About the Author

Leon Lyons is a British born, Amazon best selling author, a Psychological expert and Senior Life Coach at Mindset Mastership, based in London, England.

Leo as his known to friends used to consult global brands headquartered in central London. Although now he would say he found a more fulfilling role in life: coaching clients from around the world, changing lives for the better and when he's not travelling or surviving global pandemics, he also writes about how success can happen.

Leon Lyons has now published 5 books:

1. How To Change Habits
2. Change Mindset, Behaviour & Positive Thinking
3. How To Find Work You Love
4. Rewire Your Brain: 2 Books in 1 Master Your Mindset & Habit Hack
5. Negotiation Skills: Techniques, Tactics

These five are his first books, with many others being published within weeks. Therefore please also follow his Amazon author profile for future updates.

Here at Mindset Mastership, we help you understand what human behavior really is, and how to maximise your full potential. Whether you are stuck in business, lifestyle, dating or social life; we are here to coach and mentor you to achieve results. We have trained many clients across the globe to make radical changes to their thinking, behavior and mindset.

We are in the changing lives business.

© **Copyright 2021 by (United Arts Publishing, England.) - All rights reserved.**

This document is geared towards providing exact and reliable information in regards to the topic and issue covered. The publication is sold with the idea that the publisher is not required to render accounting, officially permitted, or otherwise, qualified services. If advice is necessary, legal or professional, a practised individual in the profession should be ordered.

- From a Declaration of Principles which was accepted and approved equally by a Committee of the American Bar Association and a Committee of Publishers and Associations.

In no way is it legal to reproduce, duplicate, or transmit any part of this document in either electronic means or in printed format. Recording of this publication is strictly prohibited and any storage of this document is not allowed unless with written permission from the publisher. All rights reserved.

The information provided herein is stated to be truthful and consistent, in that any liability, in terms of inattention or otherwise, by any usage or abuse of any policies, processes, or directions contained within is the solitary and utter responsibility of the recipient reader. Under no circumstances will any legal responsibility or blame be held against the publisher for any reparation, damages, or monetary loss due to the information herein, either directly or indirectly.

Respective authors own all copyrights not held by the publisher.

The information herein is offered for informational purposes solely, and is universal as so. The presentation of the information is without contract or any type of guarantee assurance.

The trademarks that are used are without any consent, and the publication of the trademark is without permission or backing by the trademark owner. All trademarks and brands within this book are for clarifying purposes only and are the owned by the owners themselves, not affiliated with this document.

Join Our Personal Self-Growth Power Group

To help reinforce the learning's from our books, I strongly suggest you join our well-informed powerhouse community on Facebook.

Here, you will connect and share with other like-minded people to support your journey and help you grow.

>>>Click here to join Our Personal Growth Support Group <<<

https://www.facebook.com/mindsetmastership

Mental Toughness

By Leon Lyons

Mindset Mastership,

London, United Kingdom 2021

Dedicated to my ever loving self-growth hackers at

https://www.facebook.com/mindsetmastership

Table of Contents

Chapter 1: MEANING OF MENTAL TOUGHNESS.................................. 1

Chapter 2: HOW TO BECOME MENTALLY STRONG.......................... 11

Chapter 3: MENTAL TOUGHNESS USED BY ATHLETES IN SPORTS ... 30

Chapter 4: MENTAL TOUGHNESS EXERCISES 47

Chapter 5: UPLIFT YOUR MENTAL ENERGY.. 69

Chapter 6: PREVENT PROCRASTINATION.. 77

Chapter 7: BOOST YOUR PRODUCTIVITY 85

Chapter 8: DECISION MAKING.. 93

Chapter 9: ELIMINATE NEGATIVE THINKING 100

Chapter 10: SOLID SELF-CONFIDENCE 107

Chapter 11: REPROGRAM YOUR MIND 114

Chapter 12: DEVELOP EVERLASTING SELF-ESTEEM 122

Chapter 13: INSTANT MOTIVATION 128

Chapter 14: QUICK PROBLEM-SOLVING.. 139

Chapter 15: THINKING CLEARER, SMARTER & FASTER.................... 149

Chapter 16: ACHIEVING FRUITFUL EFFECTIVENESS......................... 155

Chapter 17: GREATER EFFICIENCY 162

CONCLUSION 169

REFERENCES 173

Chapter 1: MEANING OF MENTAL TOUGHNESS

Some folks seem to have everything. They are the ones with good jobs, the perfect bodies, and the best lives. They dare to get up and go to the gym every morning. Their belief in themselves is unshakeable. They go ahead and do it regardless of how they feel when they want to get anything done. They appear to most of us as god-like.

OK, so I just slightly exaggerated. No-one has an entirely perfect life. In contrast, some of us are getting pretty close. What separates the majority of those lucky folks? What about them is it that draws success after success, chance after opportunity? You'll have discovered that these great people also have the extraordinary ability to remain positive and stoic even when everything around them begins to unravel. The first secret to mental toughness, as simple as it sounds, is understanding and embracing the ability to make choices and how that power can shape our lives. They do so because they never lack the essential tools for mental toughness. Because mental discipline is the baseline, it is the mental toughness that takes you right to the end.

Going further, have you ever wondered how those who work and live in harsh conditions continue to do so without quitting? Some even seem to love that challenge! You've probably heard about teams of Special Ops spending weeks in near-impossible missions or adventurers trekking into cold and rainy climates for months on end.

The need for self-discipline today is as critical as ever, if not more so than ever. You see, discipline is empowering, although it is unintuitive. Self-discipline empowers us to pursue what we want: the attainment of our objectives and the achievement of an exciting and enlivening life. On the other hand, a lack of self-discipline leaves us to succumb to futile and harmful urges that toss our lives in a direction we don't want. As Jim Rohn said, "we all have one of two things to suffer: the discomfort of discipline or the discomfort of regret."

Many exceptional people lead lives of a particular kind of deep focus and concentration. For example, in the Zen tradition, the average day in a Buddhist monk's life mainly consists of prayer and meditation. They abandon the temptations of the external world and focus on the highest level of emotional development. They are the most successful CEOs and the religious equivalents of Sporting gymnasts. How is it that they are so motivated? What drives them? The solution to all of these questions is one word-mental toughness.

You see, this isn't about luck at all. Indeed, some people are born with genes that make them look better or happier than the average person. But what elevates a regular Joe or Jane to the level of a superhero is a super-sharp focus, determination, and the ability to continue when everyone else has left. These are the secrets you'll learn in this book.

The concept of mental toughness has offered us a truly remarkable journey and experience. As explored in this book, what started as a small-scale intellectual experience has developed into a truly global trend. Many mental toughness techniques have proven valuable and worthwhile in most industries. What has evolved is the attribution of a personality trait that seems to be extremely important in considering individual and organizational performance, well-being, and positive behaviour development. All of these are critical in enabling people to deal with the stresses and demands of modern life.

The first question is;

What is Mental Toughness?

We define mental toughness as the quality that largely determines how people handle challenges, stressors, and pressure effectively, regardless of the prevailing circumstances. It's essential to have a clear definition of mental toughness so that everyone can look at the concept from their perspective.

One of the first moves in the model's creation and introduction to the outside world has been to create a clear, usable, and reasonable concept of mental toughness. Most of the remainder will benefit from that solid base.

Interestingly, some do not like the term mental toughness, although this is beginning to diminish as it becomes better understood and used more often. For better or worse, psychologists and practitioners in the different fields we work in have accepted for the present time that' mental toughness' is the right and proper term for what we are about to define.

This book explains and updates everything that has emerged from researching and applying the model and measure. It is written with a view to two audiences. One consists of psychology students who wish to learn about the concept, how it works, the data, and how it applies to the rest of psychological thought. The other comprises practitioners looking to understand it well enough to make effective use of it in their work. We've written the book as much as we can to be available to both audiences.

The second question is,

'Does it Exist in Reality? Can it be measured?'

The short answer is we believe there is mental toughness, and we have strong evidence to support that view. In turn, we have developed the ability to assess mental toughness usefully. This book provides a longer and more thoughtful answer to those questions.

Too much popular psychology is based solely on an individual's subjective point of view—the person often emerges as some kind of guru. There's a lot of 'Cod Psychology' out there. Much of it is based on faith: clinicians follow these 'forms' and 'approaches' based on the flimsiest proof—and sometimes no facts whatsoever.

'Can I grow mental toughness?'

We hope it can. A lot of practice in the world of sports suggests that is the case. Is it Nature or Nurture? Evidence in this book shows that mental toughness has a clear genetic link. Some people are born tough, as everybody suspects. New studies relating to brain structure affirm this aspect of design.

Nevertheless, standards of mental toughness will shift. In most of this book, I have presented techniques that can help develop mental toughness. They are sculpted from many applied psychology fields. We have asked experts to provide chapters in relaxation, attention control, and fatigue that help explain the processes involved.

'Is that helpful?'

The technical aspects are first. The chapters in this book include information about these. A different way to look at this discussion is to think about how the measure model was used and whether it helped us understand why some people perform better than others. Secondly, an equally important consideration was whether the instrument's use in applied settings has been effective. Many subtitles have been included in the book to address some of those questions. We hope you find them helpful.

The Misconceptions of Mental Toughness:

- Misconceptions 1: The idea that everyone should be mentally tough

Some people are mentally tougher than others. We would argue that mentally tough people are better able to cope with high-pressure conditions. Consequently, they tend to be better at school, at jobs, in competitive sports, and so on, and are likely to succeed in work assessment systems.

However, it should be noted that mental toughness is the opposite of mental sensitivity and not mental weakness. A mentally tough person is going to deal with stress, pressure, and challenge by not allowing it to get to them.' It's colloquially' water off the back of a duck.' A mentally sensitive person feels the effect of stress, pressure, and defeat and will' get to them' and feel the consequent reaction. Somehow, they'll be unhappy.

A structured society requires a combination of the tough and the sensitive. Identifying an extremely successful yet keen professional sportsperson is quite tricky, just as identifying a tough-minded artist can be equally tricky.

Please be aware that this does not imply that the psychologically tough are not emotionally intelligent, whatever that might mean. Emotional Intelligence (EI) characterizes a different kind of sensitivity-EI people are susceptible to what is going on in society around them and how others respond to what they are doing. Emerging evidence suggests mental toughness and emotional intelligence can go hand in hand and often does.

While it may be generally true that the mentally unbreakable seems to have a better deal in life, they often receive more. They are more likely to be promoted. They are more likely to be substantially successful, all we say here is that sensitive people find it more challenging to cope with life's stressors and pressures. They are more likely to show some of the adverse effects of being unable to cope with life changes and often suffer from depression and anxiety.

It is also clear that in dealing with the world as they find it, this book's strategies can be beneficial for everyone—the mentally vulnerable and the mentally tough. Some people are keen to be tough. Others want to live as they are, but they also wish to a toolkit of abilities to tackle those circumstances that prove challenging. There are many people who, on their terms, are successful in life but are mentally sensitive and not mentally tough.

Mental toughness provides an advantage in education, but it is certainly not the only thing for everyone, or even necessarily the main thing. Measuring mental toughness enables teaching staff to provide adequate support for different kinds of people.

There are a lot of ways to look at this issue, as ever. There is an exciting economics approach that sometimes allows us to ask the same question and obtain two different but helpful answers. Economists will discuss macroeconomics (the big picture) and microeconomics (the particular).

So we can ask a worldwide question- 'should we have a tougher mental society?' As stated above, we might conclude that we would love a balanced society, but we might argue, generally in one path or another, for a slight shift to secure an acceptable balance. A more specific question about our kids or our colleagues at work might be: would I also want them to be more mentally tough? We might know that they're likely to get a better deal in life and that they're likely to achieve more. However, while remaining comparatively mentally sensitive, we also know that they can lead a good and fulfilling life, and we know we can support them in this.

- Misconception 2: We are only interested in achievement at work or in sports

We are both attracted to performance enhancement, and it can be easy to assume that this is only linked to production, revenue, bonuses, wages, and qualifications. These are very important in many situations, but we are concerned with a much broader comprehension of performance. As economists talk about creating and distributing wealth, they generally speak in their most general sense of money. Wealth is the sum of all that adds to health and contentment.

One focus in our mental toughness training programs is the importance of setting goals. This might relate equally well to being your city's best dad or the happiest person. Mental toughness inherently contributes to the pursuit of success, implying that many mentally tough people are motivated to rise to the top of their careers. This isn't for everyone, though. For example, Peter once served on the fringes of international success with a professional swimmer. With much success, they worked together to develop her mental toughness. The result? She decided to stop swimming, and instead, she wanted to do something more! Just because you are great at something doesn't mean you're going to love it. By developing her mental toughness, she has been able to make better choices for herself in life.

- Misconception 3: Mental toughness is a concept that is macho-dominated by males

At first sight, this may seem true. However, it seems less accurate when you consider this statement in the light of misconception 2; mental toughness is about being all that you can be. While mentally tough individuals are, by nature competitive, they are almost always simply efficient with themselves. We are all related separately.

From the many studies we have conducted, there is unmistakable evidence that both men and women are equally tough. There may be some differences in the adopted coping systems and readiness to voice their opinions, but the fundamental core toughness emerges as identical from the study after study.

- Misconception 4: Mental tough people are not caring and individualistic

This relates to misconception 3 to some extent. Mentally tough people can operate well in teams. Most elite sportspeople play in extreme team environments, and they are tough mentally. The idea that tough people are always dominant and unsupportive is simply not the case. The product of low self-esteem and anxiety is a lot of bullying behaviour and minor sniping. If you are strong, safe in your skin, you have little need to assert your dominance by 'proving' other people's inferiority.

Chapter 2: HOW TO BECOME MENTALLY STRONG

How Strong Are You?

Many individuals tend to bounce back quickly from emotional defeats and losses, while others have a much tougher time. Are you able to pick yourself up and adjust to the situations when life throws you a curveball? Or do you feel incredibly frustrated, with little trust in your ability to manage the situation?

Not to stress if you fall into the above group. Fortunately, there are many practical methods for improving mental resilience; it is an ability that can be mastered and sharpened with training, dedication, and hard work.

When life conditions change suddenly and for the worse, like the loss of a loved one, the loss of a career, or the dissolution of a friendship, our strength is put to the test. On the other hand, such obstacles offer an incentive to rise above and return much more potent than before.

Continue reading to learn how to develop and strengthen your mental strength and cope effectively with life's challenges.

Four Cs of Mental Strength:

- Control

This is how much you think you have control over your life, including your feelings and sense of meaning. Your self-confidence can be called the control variable. To score high on the Control measure, you must be at peace in your skin and have a clear sense of self.

You can better control feelings, less likely to expose your emotional condition to others, and are less disturbed by other people's emotions. If you score low on the Control measure, you can feel as if incidents occur to you and you have no power or influence over them.

- Commitment

This is the degree to which you can concentrate and be dependable on your own. To score highly on the Commitment scale, you must set and accomplish goals regularly without being distracted. A high degree of commitment suggests that you're excellent at building effective routines and behaviours.

If you score low on the Commitment scale, you can find it hard to prioritize goals and adjust good routines and behaviours. Other individuals or conflicting interests can also easily distract you.

The Endurance component of the Mental strength concept is expressed by the Control and Commitment scales when taken together. This makes sense because being able to come back from losses necessitates an understanding of power over one's life and the desire to improve. It also necessitates concentration and the capacity to develop habits and set goals to help you return to your chosen path.

- Challenge

This metric tests how inspired and flexible you are. A high Challenge score shows that you are motivated to reach your personal best and consider challenges, transitions, and obstacles as opportunities instead of dangers; you are also prone to be adaptable and versatile. If you score low on the Challenge scale, you can interpret change as a threat and avoid innovative or challenging circumstances for fear of failing.

- Confidence

This is how secure you are in your capacity to be effective and capable; your self-confidence and trust in your ability to impact others. To score high on the Confidence scale, you must assume that you can achieve tasks effectively and that you can cope with challenges while keeping a routine and even improving your resolve. The confidence scale below implies that you're quickly affected by setbacks, and you don't believe you're capable or have any control over others.

The Confidence part of the Mental strength concept is expressed by the Challenge and Confidence scales when used together. This reflects the capacity to perceive and seize opportunities and the ability to accept and explore circumstances. This makes perfect sense as you are more likely to turn obstacles into good results if you are confident in yourself and your abilities and can effectively interact with others.

Basic Understanding

When my friend worked for the army, he found that agents required mental strength to work through long-running missions. He discovered that avoiding problems will not make them go away. He had to learn how to endure and work on problems lasting for an extended period.

Even after leaving the army, he was always surrounded by general life concerns that couldn't be ignored because they were complicated and inconvenient. He realized that the mental strength he had built in the military would still be required to conquer the new and different challenges and barriers in my life.

Most individuals misunderstand mental strength. It's also associated with a tough-guy attitude that refuses to bend as conditions shift.

But that isn't the whole picture. Mental strength refers to the capacity to control your feelings, emotions, and actions in ways that will help you excel. It's not something you're born with; it's an ability that can be mastered at any time, not just through difficult times.

"Be mindful of your thoughts; they turn into sentences. Keep an eye on your words because they become acts. Keep an eye on your actions; they will become habitual. Keep an eye on your habits; they shape your personality. Keep an eye on your personality; it will decide your fate." —The Chinese scholar Lao Tzu

First and foremost, our minds are biologically programmed to make us emotional beings. Our default response will always be emotional, no matter how strong and self-controllable we think we are. We can regulate or inhibit our feelings, so we're kidding ourselves if we believe we can influence how our mind handles emotions.

Nevertheless, you have full power over the feelings that accompany an emotion. You have a huge amount of influence over how you respond to your emotion and the circumstance that triggered it when you're in control.

Here are three psychological secrets to being mentally strong:

- Vision Clarity

Many individuals emerge from the chute with a strong sense of direction and vision for their lives. Some were not one of the fortunate few. Some pursued a generic business degree in school because they had no idea what they needed to do with their life. The first few jobs may also be unsuccessful. At a point, some are forced to ask themselves, "What do I not suck at?".

Many might be nervous about being a loser and how they would justify this to their parents at the time. Eventually, they know that most people have difficulty understanding what they want to do with their lives.

"How do you discover what is important to you?" is the bigger question you must answer. Mental strength necessitates a simple view of yourself and where you want to go in existence. It's what'll light a fire in your belly.

Not settling for mediocrity but rather doing the essential work requires patience and perseverance. What matters to each of us is distinct. However, mentally strong individuals find out what they want out of life and how they're going to get it.

"In a human's life, there are two wonderful days: the day we are born and the day we learn why." William Barclay

In the context of psychology, psychologist Mihaly Csiksgentmihalyi established the idea of flow, a state of mind in which individuals are so immersed if nothing else seems to matter. Csikszentmihalyi and his team discovered that inherently driven individuals are more inclined to be goal-oriented and appreciate challenges, contributing to higher overall satisfaction.

To make things right for you, follow these steps: When was the last time you forgot to eat because you were so focused on your work? When were you so engrossed in something that it felt like nothing else mattered? This is what it means to be in a state of flow. Consider the moments during the day, week, or month that you feel committed and fulfilled. That's the job you're excited about.

- Match Your Goals with Your Beliefs

It's time to set targets that will drive us on the right path once we've established the essential tasks. There are plenty of trainers, self-help books, and experts willing to give their professional guidance for a fee when it comes to setting goals. As long as the cash keeps flowing in, the results are assured.

When we have big goals, it can be challenging to know where to start. Alternatively, we can begin with everything and ignore the fact that life is unpredictable. As a consequence, when we fail to reach a target, we feel guilty, leading to responses like "I'll begin again next week."

According to psychologists, individuals who crave goals that fulfill their fundamental beliefs are more likely to persist and not give up. Beliefs are things that are more important than yourself. They're about more than just enjoyment and transient pleasures.

"Writing a stated mission isn't something you do on the spur of the moment. On the other hand, your stated mission becomes your framework, the strong representation of your values and beliefs. It becomes the yardstick from which you judge the rest of your life." —Stephen Covey, author of "The 7 Habits of Highly Successful People."

We're blue-flamers ready to take on the universe once we're out of bed. We're young, athletic, and full of energy. That helps for a while. However, if our ambitions aren't satisfying us, we'll slow down as we reach middle age.

Today, it's the new generation of people who are giving us a run for our money. Guess who'll get run over if the enthusiasm is lacking?

How to make things right for you: Everybody has specific beliefs, so you must search deep to find the ones that will contribute to your personal growth and intimate friendships.

They contrast sharply with extrinsic incentives such as cash, status, and celebrity. Make some adjustments to incorporate your beliefs further into your everyday life if none of your ambitions match what is most important to you in life.

- Cultivate a Good Mindset

Our mind is a never-ending chatterbox. We talk to ourselves at a rate of 300-1,000 words a minute, according to estimates. Since our mind's job is to keep us alert to the danger ahead, it gets alarmed when we're faced with the strange. Your brain doesn't realize that not all new and unusual things are a threat to your life. "Nothing in the world can prevent a man with the appropriate mental attitude to accomplish his goal; nothing in the world can help a man with the wrong mental attitude." Thomas Jefferson

Martin Seligman, a psychologist, is credited with developing the science of positive thinking. He believes that acquired optimism, like mental strength, is a mentality that can be built and nurtured. Our explanatory approach, according to Seligman, is the things we tell ourselves whenever terrible things happen. Permanence, Pervasiveness, and Personality (also known as the 3 P's) are the three components he describes.

A skeptic (or worrier) tells himself or herself that the negative thing is:

- It will last for a very long time. ("This isn't going to change.")

- Applies to all. ("It's still like this.")

- Is it not their fault? ("I'm not very good at this.")

A good thinker (or idealist) assures themselves that the negative thing:

- Is available for a short period. ("It happens now and then, but it's not a big deal.")

- Isn't common and has a particular cause. ("It won't be a problem if the demand changes.")

- They aren't to blame. ("It just wasn't my day.")

To make this work for you, follow these steps: Note the 3 P's and turn the tables the next time you're faced with a challenge or stumbling block.

- Don't think of a stumbling block as permanent; instead, think of it as temporary.

- Instead of being a pervasive and inevitable stumbling block, it is a one-of-a-kind case.

- Cultivate an it's-not-all-my-fault mentality instead of personalizing the issue and making it all about you.

You should train yourself to be a positive thinker that is mentally tough over time. Nevertheless, Seligman cautions against observing life via rose-tinted lenses. He argues that idealists (optimists) will misrepresent the truth in a self-serving manner, whereas worriers (pessimists) perceive reality more accurately.

Don't wait for a daunting circumstance to bring your mental strength to the test; incorporate these techniques now to be prepared for whatever comes your way.

Qualities of Mentally Strong People

We exist in tumultuous times. There are no assurances, and the future is more unpredictable than it has ever been. To cope in this troubled world, we must learn to accept confusion and control our emotions. Mentally strong people have cultivated these two forms of thinking. Below are qualities found in mentally strong people:

- Mentally strong individuals are adaptable in their thought and responsive to new information. They don't cling to old ways if they don't seem genuine or essential anymore.
- Mentally strong individuals encounter anxiety but do not allow it to deter them from advancing. Going forward can be terrifying and disturbing, but mentally strong individuals know that each challenge provides them with more strength. Staying afraid will not help you transcend your restricting

worldview. It keeps them grounded and solid. It takes courage to go against the grain, speak up, and stand out in the face of opposition and criticism to evolve as an individual and test the boundaries. Often our confused reasoning is to blame for the bulk of our problems. We learn by watching our parents and other influential people in our lives. We obtain information from culture and the media. Not all we experience is true or healthy. Therefore, It pays to be a critical thinker, willing to determine facts for yourself before deciding whether or not to believe anything.

- Mentally strong people recognize themselves. They refuse to let anyone tell them who they are, whether they are competent or what is and isn't realistic in their lives. Mentally strong individuals make their own choices and respect their views rather than others' opinions. The bulk of our suffering derives from the contrast between how we perceive life and how it is. The expression "It wasn't supposed to be like this" is one that most of us have used at some stage in our lives. Acceptance of one's current condition will make all the difference. Give up the resistance and deal with the situation as it is. Just because things don't go as expected doesn't mean all is lost. Consider this: maybe the way things are now are the way they are for a cause or a higher purpose.

- Mentally strong individuals don't stress about being happy all of the time. Happiness can creep up on us when we're least expecting it. It may also be momentary. A minor incident, such as smiling with a partner or dancing in the street, causes a chemical release of endorphins and increased serotonin. Happiness is unique to each person, not something that can be generalized. Who has the authority to tell you that your definition of pure pleasure is sucking pumpkin seeds in your shed on a rainy day? Be focused and mindful of what makes you happy, but don't obsess about it. Pursuing it just makes it more elusive. When it comes to coping with a particular situation or scenario, feelings are more important than the circumstance itself. The standard of our lives is primarily determined by how we view a problem. We can either allow ourselves to be enslaved by harmful negative thinking or motivate ourselves and encourage mental strength by fostering a positive mindset. I know it's easier said than done, but it's well worth the effort.
- Mentally strong individuals have potent minds and do not obey the crowd unconsciously. They violate the rules (but not the law), but they know what is right and wrong.
- Mentally strong individuals know that hate and anger do not damage those who are despised. They serve to irritate the hater. Animals and humans are characterized by their ability

to empathize and understand one another, and we can use this capability to make our lives simpler. Being judgmental is toxic and can contribute to prejudice. Maintain an open mind and note that the majority of folks make mistakes. Try not to say the worst of anyone all of the time. This influences you and your faith in the world, not on the people you hate.

- Ultimately, mentally strong individuals assume total responsibility for their current condition. They know that their past decisions, emotions, and behaviors have brought them to this point. They don't hold it against others because they, too, have taken decisions, even though they were passive ones. For instance, blaming an ex-partner for all your issues when you still remained with them on a subconscious or fearful level. You have more control than you are aware of. Allowing self-doubt and restricting self-beliefs to prevent us from being true to ourselves dilute our strength. Be secure in yourself, loving, compassionate, and respectful of others, and make your own decisions about the world.

Strategies to Improve and Enhance Mental Strength

As we've seen, mental strength is something that can be enhanced over one's life, not something that is fixed at birth. We'll look at a variety of mental strength methods and techniques in the parts below.

- Learning new skills

Acquiring new skills can help create endurance by establishing a sense of accomplishment and expertise, all of which may be useful during difficult times and growing one's self-esteem and problem-solving abilities.

The person will decide the skills that must be learned. Many people, for instance, can profit from developing cognitive skills like working memory or attention control, which will help them perform better in daily situations. Others may benefit from competency-based learning to learn new hobby activities.

Learning new skills in a community environment has the added advantage of offering social support, which helps create resilience.

- Setting Goals

The ability to set goals, build implementable steps to accomplish those goals, and implement all leads to stamina and mental strength growth. Goals may be big or small, and they can be for your physical health, mental well-being, job, finances, faith, or something else. Goals requiring the development of new skills would reap double benefits. Training to use an instrument or learning a new language is two examples.

According to several studies, setting and working for goals that are bigger than oneself, such as religious participation or working for a purpose, can help improve mental strength. This can give you a greater sense of mission and connection, which can help in tough times.

- The exposure that can be regulated

Regulated exposure is a method for helping people conquer their fears by gradually exposing them to anxiety-provoking circumstances. According to a study, this can help people become stronger, particularly when it includes learning new skills and setting goals — a triple gain.

For instance, public speaking is a valuable life skill and a source of anxiety for many people. Individuals who are scared of public speaking should set goals that require managed exposure to enhance or learn this ability. They can start with a small audience of one or two individuals and gradually expand their audience as time goes on.

This form of the action plan may be started by an individual or created with a qualified cognitive behavioral therapy counselor. Good activities can improve self-esteem, flexibility, and competence, which can help challenge circumstances.

- Make Connection

Our ties to family, colleagues, and society will enable us to be stronger. Good relationships with individuals who care for you and listen to your issues will allow us to regain hope during tough times. Similarly, helping others in their time of need can be immensely beneficial to us and enhance our sense of mental strength.

- Don't think of emergencies as insurmountable barriers.

We do not influence the external events that arise around us, but we do have control over how we respond to them. There will always be problems in life, but it is vital to look past whatever challenging circumstance you face and note that things will improve. When you cope with challenging situations, pay attention to the subtle ways in which you might already be feeling better.

- Understand that transition is an inevitable part of life.

According to common opinion, the only constant in life changes. Specific objectives can no longer be achievable or realizable as a result of trying situations. Accepting what you can't improve frees you up to concentrate on the aspects you have power over.

- Make progress toward your objectives.

Although it's crucial to set long-term, big-picture objectives, it's also vital to make sure they're achievable. Taking small, tiny steps allows us to accomplish our targets and work toward them daily. Every day, strive to take one little step closer to your target.

- Make a decision.

Rather than ignoring challenges and pressures and assuming they can go away on their own, try to take decisive action wherever possible.

- Look for ways to learn more about yourself.

Tragedies may also contribute to substantial personal development and learning. Living through a traumatic experience can improve our self-esteem and sense of self-worth, reinforce our ties, and teach us a lot about ourselves. Some individuals that have faced hardships have shared a deeper spirituality and a stronger appreciation for life.

- Develop a good self-perception.

Working to boost your self-confidence will help you escape challenges and develop strength. When it comes to problem-solving and trusting your judgment, getting a good view of yourself is important.

- Retain a sense of perspective.

Whenever things get rough, bear in mind that something might be a lot worse; try not to exaggerate things. When coping with stressful or traumatic incidents, it is beneficial to maintain a long-term outlook to cultivate mental strength.

- Maintain a good attitude.

We are less likely to find a solution whenever we concentrate on a thing's negative aspects and remain afraid. Maintain a positive, upbeat attitude and foresee a positive result rather than a negative one. Visualization is a method that can be useful in this regard.

- Look after yourself.

Self-care is an essential strategy for developing mental strength because it keeps your body and brain in good shape so you can handle difficult situations as they come up. Taking good care of yourself entails paying close attention to your personal needs and emotions, as well as participating in enjoyable and relaxing activities. Physical activity is also an excellent form of self-care.

- Additional resilience-building strategies may be beneficial.

To different individuals, building mental strength can mean different things. Writing things down, gratitude exercise, meditation, and other spiritual practices can help specific individuals reclaim their hope and resolve.

Chapter 3: MENTAL TOUGHNESS USED BY ATHLETES IN SPORTS

This chapter is dedicated to athletes or those who wish to develop the robust mental toughness needed for career success. Take a look at the top mental strength tips I have provided in this chapter to help you develop and use your mental strength.

When it comes to athletics, mental toughness is just as critical as physical health for players. Even the best athletes will succumb under pressure, so mental preparation is an important skill to have. One way to put it is that "when the going gets tough, the tough get going. According to a sports psychologist, " Mental toughness is "the potential to regularly perform toward the top range of your talent and ability irrespective of competitive situations," is "the ability to consistently perform toward the upper range of your talent and skill regardless of competitive circumstances."

An increasing number of athletes are trying to develop their mental strength and physical fitness habits, thanks to the growing world of sports psychology. Here, we look at some of the most famous sporting mental breakdown cases and how we can benefit from them.

There is a fine line to be drawn between mentally strong athletic achievement and under-pressure failure. "To put it plainly," Dr. John Bartholomew, an associate professor in the Department of Kinesiology and Health Education, says, "sport psychology explains the psychological variables connected with athletic activity."

There are many examples of athletes who have come so close to winning but have mentally failed at the last moment. Here, I will take you through some of the most popular sporting moments where mental pressure becomes too much and the experts' take on the situation, and some top guides to help you manage your mental game.

Last Minute Sports Mishaps

A great athlete, golfer Jean Van de Velde, was defeated by a last-minute mishap. On his way to winning the 1999 British Open at Carnoustie in Scotland, the Frenchman required a double-bogey to win the tournament. He had birdied the 18th hole in the preceding two sessions, but the misery was on the way.

Van de Velde's first shot was a catastrophe, narrowly missing the water. Situations quickly got worse when the golfer hit a shot towards the green that hit the grandstand and sent him 50 yards backward. A tired third shot got stuck in the rough and flew back into the water, capping off a sudden series of errors. Van de Velde removed his shoes and socks to find his way out of disaster. The difference between athletic glory and notoriety is razor-thin, and the margin for error shrinks with each passing year. There's a story of psychological self-destruction for any sporting legend who keeps their nerve to stage a spectacular recovery. Also, the most focused rivals have succumbed to unwelcome pressure. After leading 8-0, Steve Davis reportedly lost the 1985 World Snooker Championship final to Dennis Taylor on the last frame's black ball. Despite remaining concentrated enough to win six other championships, he was unable to do this. Jana Novotna's spectacular collapse in the 1993 Wimbledon final, after leading 2-1 to Steffi Graf, was so painful that she sobbed on the Duchess of Kent's shoulder during the award ceremony.

Psychology of Sports

With the stakes for sporting victory at an increasing rate high and increased public criticism, relief is thankfully on the way for athletes under intense pressure. Sports psychology is a rapidly evolving science that provides athletes with mental and emotional assistance to help them deal with their sports strength areas such as self-belief, focus, and intense pressure management. Sports psychology improves an athlete's mental endurance for long periods of immense focus while also boosting their confidence.

The Dutch psychologist Geir Jordet discovered that the athletes' amount of pressure increases as a game progresses. According to his findings, athletes may only overcome their anxieties of failure by practicing their entire routine ahead of time and planning their thoughts before each kick.

Rachel Foxwell, a psychologist based in the United Kingdom, concurs with Jordet's assessment of increasing fears and lowering athletes' confidence due to increased pressure. She believes that this can be extended to other sports besides football.

Sports psychology is a rising trend that intends to get athletes to fight through the tension of their game rather than being impacted by the sound of the people or even the size of an imposing competitor,' she says. 'Psychology can certainly teach you how to overcome your sense of failure; it just takes a lot of mental strength. Athletes must learn to concentrate on their target, planning each kick or shot one at a time and ignoring the crowd and fatigue.' This, I believe, is something that sports psychology can teach.'

Paul Dent, a London-based sports psychologist who has worked with the Great Britain hockey team members, agrees that the present must be prioritized. He said 'The task is to concentrate on what you're doing, to have a limited attentional concentration on the here-and-now, and not on the fact that thousands of people are watching (which is a vast attentional concentration) or the consequences of missing out (the future).

'Mental toughness comes from experience and is defined as the capacity to do those as mentioned earlier in the most complicated of circumstances. Andy Scott, a California businessman, won the gold medal for completing the most challenging biking trail in Colorado in under nine hours. Even better, he scaled Mount Tyndall, California's highest peak at 14000 feet (4267 meters).

He claims that his family's opinions and readiness enable him to achieve success in such ultra high-altitude circumstances. He also mentions that the first obstacle is realizing that your mind will begin to tell you that you're exhausted and want to withdraw. Still, once you get past that, you can attain a flow state in which you're entirely focused on the present moment, pondering on nothing else, and your body produces its peak output. If you can get past the initial fear reaction, you'll be well on your way to success.

Boost Your Mental Toughness at Will

Several athletes search for answers about how to become "mentally tough," but few know how to develop it. Worse still, several athletes and coaches have no idea what mental toughness is or how it can improve their success.

Professional athletes and Olympians extol the virtues of mental toughness preparation, saying that mental toughness allowed them to accomplish great athletic success.

"Sport is so much about mental toughness. It's drilling down. It's doing everything you have to help a team win," said Tom Brady, quarterback of the New England Patriots.

Athletes' worst threat is an absence of mental toughness. Athletes who lack mental toughness relinquish, give in, tank the match, and offer less.

Your level of mental toughness is directly proportional to your athletic performance. To be mentally tough, you must be able to go above and beyond what most athletes do.

Demystifying the Idea of Mental Toughness

Many athletes assume mental toughness is something you are born with. You either have mental toughness, or you don't, according to a common opinion. And you won't be able to compete in your sport because you were not born with the mental toughness gene.

It doesn't have to be that manner, though. You are correct that mental toughness development is needed for success, but you are entirely incorrect, thinking you cannot get mentally stronger.

Some athletes, such as those who have dealt with hardships in their lives and are used to recovery, tend to be more mentally challenging than others. I'm speaking about Greg Norman and Michael Jordan, to name a couple of athletes who excelled in the face of difficulties.

Mental toughness requires the ability to cope with hardship. Mental toughness is a mindset, and you are the only one who can shape your attitude.

You will debunk the manner you think about yourself or your potential to thrive if you are the one who is responsible for your beliefs. By altering your mindset, you will change your feelings about yourself, transforming how you behave, practice, and perform.

Mental toughness is a mindset, not a typical characteristic, but it is also a habit.

In sports, mental toughness isn't something you take out of your back pocket when the game is down to the final seconds or when a 3-foot putt is needed to win a game, or even when you're up to bat in the ninth inning with the bases filled.

Mental toughness necessitates a steadfast attitude to the sport's difficulties. You must concentrate, prepare, and develop your mental toughness habit regularly.

You will perform at the peak of your physical abilities when mental toughness preparation becomes a habit. You're also more prepared to deal with difficulties, intervention, and challenging situations without losing confidence or inspiration.

Mental toughness is similar to physical fitness in that the more you exercise, the fitter you get. If you stop working out, your fitness level decreases. If you don't take care of your mental health daily, your mental toughness will deteriorate.

In other words, mental toughness isn't a one-size-fits-all proposition. Mental toughness comes in different ways. This is excellent news because mental toughness preparation will help all athletes.

You will find a noticeable change in your results as your mental toughness levels improve.

"Mental toughness is as physical as four is to one." Bobby Knight

8 Mental Toughness Qualities:

Mentally tough athletes:

- Look for a solution rather than an excuse

Mentally tough athletes don't give excuses when events don't go their direction. Rather than accusing others, they accept responsibility for their actions, return to the drawing board, put things right, and strive again.

- Adapt

Rather than doing things the same way they've always done them, mentally tough athletes discover creative ways to test themselves and push themselves to their peak. Mentally tough athletes know that what they did yesterday helped them get to where they are now. However, something needs to be done today to get them to where they need to be in the future.

- Concentrate their attention on things that can make them perform better

Mentally tough athletes concentrate on what they can manage. Mentally tough athletes don't focus on the past, feel very sorry for themselves, or think about distractions that aren't under their control. Mentally tough athletes reflect on what they should do right now to solve output problems and improve their success chances.

- Consider the past as nothing more than a valuable archive of history

Mentally tough athletes grow from their past and other people's mistakes, then let go of the past and move on. Mentally tough athletes view the past as mental preparation for potential success. Mentally tough athletes aren't characterized by their mistakes, faults, or losses; instead, these events reinforce their determination.

- Take chances

Mentally tough athletes recognize the sense of failure keeps them from completely dedicating themselves to their sport and striving for excellence. Mentally tough athletes search for ways to drive themselves outside of their comfort zones. Mentally tough athletes tackle difficulties with excitement rather than apprehension and anxiety. Mentally tough athletes refuse to be mediocre and realize that while they may sometimes miss the mark, it is worth taking the risk to accomplish amazing things.

- Persist in the face of setbacks

Mentally tough athletes are never overwhelmed by setbacks. Mentally tough athletes know that failure is yet another step on the path to success. Mentally tough athletes believe that loss is not the end of the world and never give up on their goals.

- Aim for success rather than perfection

Mentally strong athletes have a goal in mind, but their emphasis is on the steps required to reach that goal. Mentally tough athletes realize that peak success is a marathon, not a sprint. Each action they take gets them closer to their primary goal. They are unafraid of making errors, do not aspire for perfection, drive themselves to the full, and strive for everyday change.

Mentally tough athletes know that they will make mistakes in life and that these failures are both acceptable and vital stepping stones on their road to success.

- Be concerned about their strengths and abilities

Mentally tough athletes don't strive to impress others or criticize other athletes' success. They concentrate on themselves, their skills, developing themselves, putting their game plan into effect, and reaching the objectives they set for themselves.

- Talent can be underestimated

Thousands of talented athletes are never able to hit the top of their sport. In reality, 75% of all teen athletes drop out of sports, not due to a lack of skill but due to a loss of enjoyment in sports and a lack of mental toughness to perform at higher levels.

Without mental toughness, skill is useless. When it comes to regular results, preparation can be average. Average ability combined with mental toughness, on the other hand, helps good athletes to achieve greatness.

"The margins of victory are commitment and mental toughness." Russell, Bill

Champion Level Mental Toughness

Build a mental toughness habit – Discover ways to develop your mental toughness during training periods. Rather than ignoring them, look for ways to strengthen your mental game. Then, one by one, support the mental toughness's weaker aspects.

When you feel tired, keep going for another five minutes. Perform one more session than you believe you are capable of. Face challenges with resolve rather than resentment. Make a consistent dedication to mental toughness. Make a deliberate decision on how you will react to adversity.

Mental toughness is dictated by your habits, which you regulate. It's important to note that mental toughness is about fighting small battles regularly. If you aren't focusing on growing your mental toughness capacity behind the scenes, you can't hope to be mentally tough in championship times.

Fight and prove to yourself that you can persevere through each challenge you face on your way to achieving your objectives. Mia Hamm, a great soccer player, said, "I'm building a fire, and every time I practice, I add more fuel," I strike the match at precisely the right time."

How are you going to integrate mental toughness preparation into your game? How are you going to make it a regular habit?

Begin by applying each of the strategies provided in the later chapters of this book

Mental toughness is a set of psychological skills that include unwavering self-confidence, grit, determination, concentration, and the ability to work under immense pressure, and the capacity to adapt to physical and emotional pain.

Mental skills preparation is used in sport psychology to enable athletes to improve mental toughness. Mental skills preparation includes identifying athletes' strengths and limitations and designing a curriculum that improves key areas critical to their sport and personal needs. While every athlete's requirements are unique, many use similar techniques.

Setting goals

To achieve a good result, athletes can use a range of goal-setting techniques. They will set performance and process targets and a result target of winning a medal or being among the high performers.

Self-referenced performance goals can include the purpose of setting a new personal record. Method goals center athletes' attention on the technological elements that are needed for success. They're the "hows" and "forms" of achieving a desired result or success standard.

For instance, a long jump athlete to receive a medal and land a spectacular jump effectively may move his focus to the aspects within the jump that he understands he can — and must — do to land every jump effectively. This will improve his self-assurance and reduce any disturbing feelings of defeat or things he can't manage, including his rivals. For certain athletes, concentrating on the result may detract from their results and make them their own worst enemy.

Nathan Chen, the American figure skater who overcame a catastrophic short program to complete a world-record six quad jumps in the free skate at the Winter Olympics, has spoken about the "mental energy" required for each jump in his free skate program. Nathan Chen of the United States, who broke the world record with six quad jumps in the men's free skate at the Pyeongchang Olympics, says he mentally breaks down almost every jump before performing.

Self-talk

Self-efficacy is an athlete's unwavering belief in their ability to overcome an obstacle. It is, without a doubt, the foundation of any fantastic performance. Self-talk is a technique that can improve self-efficacy and performance.

The inner conversation we make with ourselves is known as self-talk. We have over 50,000 thoughts in a single day. Thoughts can influence an athlete's confidence. While it's extremely difficult for an athlete to keep records of all of their thoughts in a single day, they can practice good self-talk. Reassurances of their power and trigger words that boost them up or relax their nerves are examples of this form of self-talk. Straightforward reassurances of where their concentration should be and what they have to do can be included.

At the top of the hill or walking out onto the center ice, good athletes successfully control their emotions, ensuring they are their own closest buddy. Finally, this method has the amazing potential to make an athlete feel confident, in command, and ready to take on any challenge.

Cassie Sharpe of Canada wins gold in the women's ski halfpipe at the 2018 Winter Olympic Games in Pyeongchang. Sharpe and other athletes often view their whole routines moments before beginning, including spinning their bodies to mimic the moves.

Visualization

Visualization is a complicated ability to master. However, when done, it allows an athlete to visualize themselves conducting their skill from beginning to end as if they were doing it in near real-time.

Visualizing is the process of simulating the actual action that an athlete wants to perform while using all of their senses. What's more amazing is that, with enough practice, the practice muscles will perform in the same order and level in actual situations. One of the mental skills that could be most relied on as an athlete is visualization.

To prepare for the tournament, you should spend many hours visualizing what you need to do and the way you have it to feel. You can even play out worst-case scenarios in your head, feeling the immense pressure and distress and practicing your appropriate reactions. When it comes time to compete, you automatically feel prepared for any scenario. This is the most challenging aspect of preparation by far, but you need to perform well when it mattered most.

We watch athletes practice visualization the most in sliding games like luge and bobsleigh. The earth pull that these athletes are exposed to is hazardous to their health and restricts their skill to practice their sport physically.

Controlling Stimulation

Athletes have a sweet spot when it comes to how they want to feel when they're at their best. This is their optimum level of stimulation. A few athletes could choose to be revved up, whereas some others could choose to be so calm that you question if they even realize they're about to compete.

Successful athletes have their level of stimulation tuned in, just like an air conditioner that controls the temperature in a house. They will control it if they find themselves outside of it.

For instance, an athlete can reduce stimulation by drawing deep breaths from the diaphragm and practicing self-talk to become calmer. Athletes can also raise their stimulation level by taking shorter breaths or playing music. The most crucial part is that the athlete feels in control of their emotions.

There's no denying that mental toughness gives an athlete an edge over their opponent when it comes to high performance. Although some athletes may be born with this natural talent, it can be developed and built up. Good athletes are well conscious of the value of mental toughness. Many world-class athletes realize that enhancing mental skills is just as critical as improving physical and technological abilities.

Chapter 4: MENTAL TOUGHNESS EXERCISES

Mental Toughness Exercises Used by Athletes

Most topics on mental toughness among athletes, high school and college coaches center on modeling mental toughness, developing confidence, concentration, composure, commitment, and helping players with fear, depression, and other mental health issues. In this chapter, I will share exercises on coping with feedback, improving concentration, and some mental toughness takeaways.

- Work on mental skills daily. Mental toughness is critical in sports activities just as much as it is for professional athletes. You probably work a day job and don't have as much time as you'd like to practice or compete. As a consequence, you must make the most of your chances to change quickly. Working on your mental skills for a few minutes a day, every day, as the Champion's Mind app helps you to do, is one of the easiest ways to do this. Since mentality affects actions, the more mentally strong you are, the better your performance and the more pleasure you will have. Mental toughness is described as the ability to remain optimistic and constructive in the face of adversity. If you've had a tough day at work, it's time to put it behind you and mentally prepare for the evening match. Your mental game has the power to make all the difference. Everyone you're up against has a hectic schedule and no time to practice. You'll have a distinct advantage if you build a gold medal mentality.

- We all face distractions and stuff that irritate us at different times during the day. Reframing situations that you would usually think of negatively in a better light is one way to exercise mental toughness. Instead of seeing them as obstacles to escape, think of them as problems to resolve. Say to yourself, "This is my Olympics," and find a way to make the most of it, whether you're stuck in traffic, have a pile of work on your desk, or have a difficult workout. Turn a situation that you'd typically only want to get through into an opportunity to learn. Reflecting on how you overcame stressful situations in the past is another easy way to improve mental toughness. What did you say to yourself to lift your spirits during these difficult times? What qualities, such as dedication, bravery, and calmness, did you use to drive through and resolve whatever you were up against? Remind yourself about how strong and diligent you've been in the past the next time you face a somewhat insurmountable challenge, and then decide to demonstrate the same determination this time.

- Every technically demanding sport necessitates the use of visualization. Create a list of the techniques and moves you want to learn and the kind of athlete you want to be. Then visualize your favorite rival flawlessly executing them. Put yourself in their shoes until you have a good mental image of them doing the new moves and techniques. Then picture yourself making the moves flawlessly over and over. Visualize and feel yourself doing what you know you should do with your body in your mind. Individuals are often hurt because they are not physically or mentally equipped. Instead of seeing this as a disappointment, use it as an encouragement to do whatever you can to change your mind and body. The question you should be asking yourself is, "How can I be at my best today?" instead of "How can I stop getting wounded?" Concentrate on the process of reaching that point once you've found the answer. Be positive and definitive whenever it comes to executing these moves in competition. Trust your preparation and bear in mind all of the hard work you've put in to get here. Enjoy the opportunity to demonstrate your success, and be thankful for the chance to contend. To free your mind, draw a deep breath and say a mantra or power thinking many times, such as "Let's do this!"

- Taking a few minutes to write down all of your achievements on an index card is a perfect way to improve your self-esteem. Include the best achievements, moments when you went above and beyond, awards, and public relations. Then add in the feedback you've got from your coaches and teammates. This is no longer just a piece of postcard; it's a confidence card. You should turn to it if you're feeling nervous or uncertain of yourself. When you're setting and dreaming about goals, take a look back at your magical moments. You'll no longer have to wish or assume that you're capable of accomplishing daunting and big goals; you'll have evidence that you can. This implies that you can and can achieve your goals once more.

- To keep your athletic dual-career focused while still being mindful of the value of your dual career (such as a professional athlete or a student-athlete). It's simply about being exactly where your feet are at all times. When it's time to go to work or play with your teammates, use the act of putting on your uniform to signify that you'll be an athlete for the next few hours. And not just any competitor, but one who has won a championship. Close the door on everything else and put it in a mental locker. When you return, it will still be there. Then, at work or in training, decide to be the best employee or student you can be. It takes mindfulness, dedication, and concentration to make this distinction between your two positions. You're the type of individual who brings these qualities, as well as a competitive spirit, to everything you do. Decathlete with a world record, Dan O'Brien, was once asked how he could succeed in each of his sport's ten events. He answered that when he competed, he saw himself as a participant in whatever activity he was participating in at the time. And he was a shot putter, not a decathlete, as he threw the shot put. That's an outstanding example of being completely present and engaged. Working on your machine, for example, is a more boring illustration. When you open Microsoft Word or Excel to begin work or school assignments, you can close your internet browser and any other software so that you can completely concentrate on the work at hand. Use the same idea to your sport while still balancing your other obligations.

- Push yourself to the limit. I once overheard an experienced coach saying that unless you're working hard in training to the point where your teammates are judging you, you're probably not working hard enough. When you stretch yourself to your limits, you lead by example and set a positive standard for those around you. That's an achievement to be proud of. Your teammates will love you for it, even though they don't like you for it. To make you feel better, you can not hold back or cut yourself down. Whenever you offer your all in a match, it helps your whole squad, just as a rising tide raises all boats. So, every time you step onto the field or court, constantly give it your all. However, if it isn't simply one or two of your colleagues who are upset with your strategy, but most of them, you can talk with your coach to ensure you don't have to change something. The real problem likely is that your colleagues don't know you very well. Make it a point to ask them more questions and thank them for encouraging you to play with them. They will grow to like you and vice versa, and the issue will resolve itself.

- People often discuss breaking out of their physical comfort zones, but few recognize that we all have emotional ones as well. Begin to invite input from coaches, teammates, and those who can assist you develop as an athlete and a person. This does not extend to all criticism. If somebody is just slamming you for the sake of slamming you, you must learn to ignore them. In general, if you wouldn't take someone's opinion since they don't understand what they're talking about, you shouldn't take their critique. Clear and helpful criticism, on the contrary, will enable you to become a champion.

Saying to a teammate or coach, "I had a tough game," is one way to get it. What would you do differently if you could?" This demonstrates that you respect their input and trust them to assist you in improving. They could send you a couple of helpful tips on boosting your performance the next time around. In this way, you can redefine criticism as a welcome gift rather than a personal attack.

Mental Toughness Exercises Used by Navy Seals

In this chapter, I've summarized the exercises and methods used by various ex-SEALs down to a simple six exercises after reviewing several memoirs from various ex-SEALs. Every exercise is followed by a brief description and a real-world implementation.

- Eat the Elephant is the first exercise.

What is the safest way to eat an elephant? One bite at a time. When confronted by a tough challenge, a marathon, a pretty girl on the street, or a startup launch, we sometimes feel panic, freeze, and stop before we even get started.

The SEALs give a differentiation solution. Steadily dissect the elephant into digestible chunks, and well, you get the message. Take one small move at a time toward your target. It's cliched, but it's successful. Most super-marathoners and triathletes would be doing this. They keep their minds on the next possible target, the next level on the horizon, and don't let their thoughts drift to the entire race.

Application

Break down any overwhelming request into small, manageable targets. They can best fit into a 24-hour frame. Concentrate entirely on completing one mission at a time. Don't care about the big picture.

- Visualize Success

This one took me off balance. Basketball players increased their free-throw precision by 23% in one study by actually visualizing the free throws. Just 24% of players who attempted real free throws progressed. That's a gap of less than 1%. Yeah, that was amazing.

The attributes of a strong visualization are as follows:

1. Informative and vibrant. Using all of the senses. Consider the details. Make it as believable as you can.
2. Repetition is necessary. In your brain, run over the many play-by-play. Make it an automated operation.
3. Use of optimistic imagery. Do not imagine yourself as a loser. Instead, imagine yourself in a state of effortless performance daily.

4. Consider the consequences. Consider the effects of failure if the fortitude wanes. Watch the looks on your friends and family's faces as they read the news. Remember the torment of personal humiliation.

Using visualizations to visualize yourself thriving the next time you have a significant, stressful event coming up.

- Emotional Management

A surge of our system's major stress hormones, adrenaline, cortisol, and norepinephrine, will offer us a jolt of energy and concentration in times of tremendous stress. Nevertheless, when such hormones remain elevated for a prolonged period, we are unable to relax. We have difficulty sleeping, our motivation plummets, and our immune system suffers.

The simple solution devised by the SEALs is known as the four by four for four:

1. Inhale for 4 seconds.
2. 4 seconds of exhalation
3. Repeat for another 4 minutes.

Does this look familiar to you? Thousands of years have passed after yogis did anything similar. Our brain affects our bodies and vice versa. Simple respiration exercises will help you turn off your stress hormones and relax your system for rest.

Application

If you already meditate, this will help. However, if you don't, pause and take some slow breaths the next time you feel anxious. Before continuing with your day, best-selling author Tim Ferriss suggests pausing and taking three simple breaths.

- Nonreactivity

"Men are troubled not by things, but by their impressions of them," Epictetus. We have more influence than we know. We do not influence what happens in the world around us, but we control how we perceive it.

D.H. Xavier recounts his own "Hell Week" encounter in his book, Breaking BUD/S: How Ordinary Guys Could Become Navy SEALs. "They kicked me when I was down and out. My assumption may have been that they didn't want me there, and as a result of that assumption, I would have left. Rather, I assumed that I was unconcerned with what they said. I was confident in my ability to succeed."

Xavier uses a method I call reframing. He excludes one potential belief or ideology and replaces it with another. What may have seemed to be a negative experience becomes a positive one.

Take a good look at how you're seeing what's going on around you. When you've defined it, question it. Any negative feelings should be reframed into more positive ones. Consider "evil" incidents as a reason to get out there and better yourself.

- Small Wins

What do you do if the motivation is low? You've forgotten your wallet, it's raining, and your wife has just abandoned you. What do you do when nothing goes right, and all thing goes wrong? Attempt to think in smaller terms. Every day, try to write three things you are thankful for in your diary.

1. After a prolonged rain, the air is cool and refreshing.
2. Iced coffee with a smoky aftertaste.
3. At your local cafe, you exchange a smile with the barista.

Tiny wins raise motivation. High motivation breeds greater motivation. It provides a positive feedback loop for doing good work. If you haven't already, give it a shot. It's a lot more critical than you would expect.

- Finding Your Tribe is Strategy

Sebastian Junger writes in his book Tribe: On Homecoming and Belonging: "Human beings don't fear adversity; in reality, they flourish on it; what they don't like is not feeling needed. The practice of making people feel unneeded has been mastered in society today. It's past time for that to stop."

Junger may be onto something here. We've all heard stories of remarkable human success in the face of adversity. It's the classic case of a mother using her mind to raise a car to save her child. Human beings are social species. And we yearn for meaning in a world that may feel all too hollow at times. You will create a significant source for mental toughness if you have both — close friends and close values.

Application

Take some time to consider what gives your life meaning. That's the first step toward discovering your tribe, a group of individuals with shared interests and values. That is everything there is to it. There are six basic techniques. You've got the supplies that are needed. All that's left to do now is apply.

Mental Toughness Exercise for Entrepreneurs

- Perform a time audit.

Look back and remember how you spend the whole day. This will help you decide if your decisions are in line with your priorities and interests. We have hopes and aspirations for which we are not making any progress. Taking a step back to evaluate how you spend your time will help you readjust your actions and choices with what you want to be doing.

- Every day, write five things you're thankful for.

Note down five things you were thankful for during the day for three weeks, every night before bed. They can be small, such as having someone hold the door for you, or big, such as having a caring family. According to research, people who practice gratitude are satisfied and more grateful for their lives. This gratitude can be channeled into everyday energy, making you more efficient and positive, both desirable qualities in an entrepreneur.

- Acquire a new skill.

Attempt to learn something new. Bonus points if it's something you've always love to learn and never felt confident in your ability to do so. It's quite simple to slip into a routine where the bulk of your work is focused on implementation rather than requiring serious thought. Learning a new ability is an ideal way to exercise your brain. Plus, it will encourage you to practice something you've been considering for a long time.

- Find anyone who disagrees with a deeply held opinion of yours and discuss it with them.

We are rarely faced with questions regarding our values. While this makes it easier because we don't have to justify our positions all of the time, it also implies that we don't need to worry about why we believe what we believe. Find something on which you have firm opinions and address it with someone who has the opposite perspective.

It's a mentally relaxing activity to listen to and counter their points. You'll also come away from the interview with new insights and greater confidence in your original belief or a particular viewpoint. You must be able to think objectively and question your preconceived ideas to be a good entrepreneur. This kind of mental exercise is excellent preparation.

- Examine the circle of friends you keep.

We are an average of the five individuals with whom we spend most of our time. As a consequence, keeping track of who you spend your time with is highly beneficial. What contribution do they make to your life?

It doesn't have to be concrete, like a wealthy friend who pays for your holidays. A friend who makes you smile or makes you feel good is simply as important, if not more so, than a friend who makes you feel good. The number of individuals in your life with whom you have no valid reason to spend time would shock you.

And, by the number of people you care for but don't have enough time for. Using this audit to help you spend more time with the people you honestly fancy being around and less time with the people you do not. You'll be happier and more productive as a result of this.

- To observe how much you've changed, find a piece of yourself from the past.

It is thought-provoking to flashback on your past, whether it is an old diary note, past academic writing for a class, or even a picture. It shows how much you've improved since then. It can also act as a reminder of your core beliefs and values. Looking back will help you remember why you felt a certain way in the first place. This will also expose how you are behaving in ways that are inconsistent with your beliefs and assist you in realigning your life.

- Read

Reading is a perfect way to keep the mind sharp. It's an excellent way to learn new facts, ideas, and opinions. Furthermore, some reading, which for the most part is fiction, is simply pleasurable. It's easy to find reasons to stop reading, but even taking 15 minutes a day to do so will expand your horizons and provide you with more tools to solve problems.

- Throughout the day, listen to podcasts or audiobooks.

Between traveling, getting dressed, eating meals, and waiting, we have a considerable amount of free time every day. Allowing your mind to unwind from time to time may be helpful. But a lot of the time, the time is spent worrying about unimportant things. Listen to audiobooks or podcasts instead.

This will encourage you to benefit from other people's experiences while also keeping you updated about current events. Take advantage of the fact that getting this audio content is simpler than ever.

- Spend as much time as possible without causing your thoughts to drift.

It's challenging to keep your mind focused on the job at hand. It is, however, imperative to be able to improve this ability. It enables you to be completely present in every situation and to enjoy life to the fullest. Try to be as mindful as possible during the day.

It's perfectly natural for your mind to drift to the past or another circumstance. Only be mindful of it and attempt to get out of it. This can be exhausting psychologically, but it will pay off handsomely. You'll devote more mental resources to problem-solving and completing everyday activities if you practice complete presence.

- Try something you've never done before.

We are much more capable than we realize. You could go three days without feeding, sleep four hours a night for a week, or run ten miles the next day. Although you might say that these are more physical than mental activities, they include a mental challenge. You don't have to risk your life to challenge yourself.

Instead, consider something you've always liked to do but never felt you could. Make a solid commitment to following through with it, and then do so. Trying something and confirming to yourself that you can do it, whether it's a workout, a new diet, or a routine, is inspiring. It illustrates that everything is possible, which is a mentality that every entrepreneur requires.

Mental Toughness Exercises Used by Marines

- State Your Identity

One of the military's first things to their recruits is to strip away "self-talk" and identity. This is beneficial because many people in today's culture have a misconception of how to identify themselves. Their first stop is typically their job or place at a company. "I'm the Executive Vice President of...," she says. But who are you, in reality? When that disappears, who are you? So, regardless of the situation, who do you want to be? I ask people to put it into an "identity speech," as I like to call it. "I am a man of distinction who always respects his commitments," is mine. That is who I am, regardless of the part I am playing, and I tell myself that every day.

- Retrain the brain to think more positively and constructively.

Leadership is described as the ability to impact others, but how can you hope to impact others if you can't even influence your behavior? Self-management is one of the first things you understand as a Marine. It's often referred to as brainwashing, but it's more accurately defined as cognitive reprogramming. Start with minor improvements that can be introduced right away and work your way up. Begin small and demonstrate to yourself that you can control yourself before attempting to control others.

- Examine your thoughts.

I operated security details for Joe Lieberman, Hillary Clinton, and Benjamin Netanyahu after my time in the Marines. Consequently, I had to think about not just my actions but also the actions of other people. The experience taught me how to control my emotions. If I were driving a high-value target around in a security vehicle and somebody cut me off, I wouldn't be able to get angry or respond in any way other than to keep everybody in the car safe. Then I'd get into my car and become angry, putting others or myself in danger. I began to see how my intellectual laziness was the root of the problem. In that case, I wasn't double-checking myself. So I do now, and I'm reaping the rewards of it.

- Think targets rather than constraints.

Tell anyone not to think of a pink elephant when they're thinking of you. So, what are their thoughts on the subject? An elephant that is pink in colour. Ask a golfer not to hit the sand trap. What would happen to the ball? Through the sand trap. Setting objectives is easier if you imagine them being accomplished, and if there is any action or feeling that is hindering your success, remove it entirely.

- Empathy and recognizing the reality of others

When you don't accept their reality and want to force your truth on them, you run the risk of alienating those with whom you're working. It's necessary to understand the distinction between reality and fact. For instance, if you're coming from Mexico, arriving in a city with a temperature of 60 degrees may feel cold, which is real. If anyone else is traveling from the Arctic, it will look much warmer to them, and they will be right. If you want to persuade them of something, use evidence rather than your reality. That'll be a lot more effective.

- "Devil dog, shock troop, bloodsucking war machine, ready to fight, destroy, ready to die, but never will."

Our unit officer would order us to say our prayers each night before we went to sleep in the Marines. "Devil dog, shock troop, bloodsucking war machine, ready to fight, ready to kill, ready to die, never will," we said in our prayer. That might be unsettling to hear right now, but it transformed our outlook on how we will succeed in war. I believed I was bulletproof during my career, and I reaped the rewards of that conviction. The brain receives a large amount of information regularly, but only a tiny portion is stored. According to studies, if the mind believes anything, it will seek evidence that confirms that conviction. If you think you're bulletproof, your mind will automatically gravitate toward knowledge that will help you remain bulletproof. So believe in what you're doing, and the mind will assist you in achieving your goals.

Other Mental Toughness Exercises

Irrespective of your profession or career, the following mental toughness exercise will help you in your journey of success.

- Eliminate all extrinsic motivators.

Here are a few possibilities to consider:

1. You go to your good, cool, air-conditioned gym first thing in the morning before going to work. You arrange to meet with your fitness partner to discuss your game plan for today's session. You put on your headphones and turn up the volume on your favorite extreme metal workout playlist.
2. You come home from a long and exhausting day at work, grab a sandbag and a set of heavy kettlebells, and move out to an empty park on a scorching day. You lost your headphones at home, so there was no music to listen to, no motivational training buddy, just you. You'll have to suffer in silence for a bit.

Which of these two examples would provide you with a more successful workout? I'm sure the majority of you will prefer scenario number one. The atmosphere is ideal, you're fully rested, and your buddy is there to drive you through those final reps. But here's the crux of the matter.

Will you ever put yourself in situation number two?

Or would you prefer to be at ease?

You have to bring yourself in that dark place now and then, away from all those extrinsic motivators, and battle it out with yourself. You'd be shocked how easily those little voices in your head appear and begin nagging you.

"No one is looking, so you can take it easy..."

"Ugh, my knee ain't feeling good – I'm sure it's the old injury I can only stop..."

"Just go home."

"It's perfect if you miss one workout."

The voices are triumphant. They convince you to give up. Feeling familiar with your negative thoughts and avoiding outside distractions will make a big difference. Pay attention to them, laugh at them, and keep driving. You'll be a happier person as a result.

- Developing Healthy Habits

Mentally tough people can be very consistent. They know that inspiration ebbs and flows and that to be truly efficient, they must constantly focus on the things that matter most. They are mindful of the obstacles in their way and proceed irrespectively. And it is this trait that distinguishes the successful people from the unsuccessful.

You must build behaviors that will help you accomplish your objectives and adhere to them irrespective of how tempting it might be to stray. Without depending on your internal motivation every day, great behaviors will help you defeat the obstacles you'll face on your champion's Journey. When you prefer discomfort over comfort regularly, you create a controlled behavior that is difficult to break.

Make it a habit to charge forward and tackle the challenges ahead of you one by one. Baby steps. Good behaviors and disciplined behavior will help you grow the mental toughness you'll need for the rest of your life.

- Learn to disregard the things you can't change.

In his book The Obstacle is the Way, Ryan Holliday addresses the Stoic ethic, or the capacity to withstand discomfort or suffering without voicing emotions or moaning. The fundamental principle is that what counts is the way you respond to what comes to you. You have full control over the way you react to any circumstance.

Chapter 5: UPLIFT YOUR MENTAL ENERGY

One of the main contributors to individuals' energy levels is the mind. The advantages of maintaining a high mental energy level include satisfaction, confidence, concentration, improved resilience, enthusiasm, and efficiency, which is why learning how to improve energy when it is low can be so valuable.

Also, the subconscious has an immense impact on one's amount of physical energy. Enhanced motivation and determination also contribute to healthy eating behaviors, less procrastination, and more.

The way we think has an enormous impact on the way others view us and how we work. You appear confident whenever you feel confident. Therefore, you can function more efficiently, increasing the chance of accomplishment with everything you do when you boost your energy levels for the long term.

This chapter covers strategies s to improve your mental energy level.

Strategies to Boost Your Mental Energy

- Be grateful.

Remind yourself of the aspects of your life that you are happy or glad about. Gratitude is going to help you think more optimistically and provide you with more mental energy.

Be happy that you have a job and you are earning a wage if you're not enjoying fun currently at work. Recognize that difficulties make you better if you face challenges in every part of your life, and be happy that you don't have a miserable life.

You are reminded of what is important by being grateful. You may be angry about being held in traffic, for instance. Being grateful to see your families again will remind you of the complete irrelevance of the traffic.

- Practice Negative Visualization

Negative visualization emerged in a philosophy called Stoicism. Stoics regularly imagine, but do not think about, "worst-case scenarios."

When these scenarios are valid, negative visualization is performed to reduce the effect. It's also designed to decrease insatiability and push you to enjoy what you have.

Many of us waste our idle time dwelling on the things we like but don't have. Stoics say we'd be much better off, spending this time thinking about all the stuff we have and thinking about how much we'd miss them if they weren't ours.

- Surrounding yourself with the right individuals

Generally, human beings are social, so creating bonds makes us happy and provides us energy. Spend some time with individuals who think positively and raise capacity just by being who they are. When you're around individuals who give this kind of insight, it will make you react better to life.

Who is overly pessimistic in your life? Should you spend as much time with them as you do with yourself? What kinds of individuals do you want to spend more time with? Build a game plan for meeting such individuals or spending time with them and eliminate the negative people.

- Positive Thinking

You will feel more optimistic by sustaining positive thoughts. Mental energy would be improved by becoming more positive and confident.

A good way to start changing negative energy is to push yourself to think positively if you feel slow or stressed. Momentum has a great impact on our energy levels as the energy builds upon itself. If the levels of mental energy are decreasing, it becomes harder and harder to continue enhancing them.

In every case, concentrate on the positive energy. As they express themselves, you benefit from the opportunity—dream of what could go well, rather than worrying about what might be wrong.

- Declutter The Mind

Many individuals are busy and have a lot on their minds, which when you try to increase energy could get in the way. We are receiving information at a higher rate than ever. Declutter your mind by assigning, setting deadlines, taking notes, and maintaining a schedule.

Hold as much as you can outside of your head to stop getting it wrong and declutter your mind. For instance, if you set up a meeting with anyone, put it on your calendar so that you don't have to recall it anymore. Maintain a list of to-do tasks, as it will help you to be more aware and mindful of what you are doing at a particular time. You'll learn more about this in later chapters.

- Go outside

You will be given Vitamin D by exposing your body and eyes to sunlight, improving energy.

Moreover, during the daytime, our brains and bodies are used to being alive, and during those hours, we usually have more energy. Having exposure to sunlight informs our body that we ought to have more energy and daytime.

Takeaway: Take a quick break outside in the sun if you feel exhausted while at work.

- Have some Fun!

Do not fail to devote time to your friends and family. This provides enthusiasm and keeps you focused. It sounds counterintuitive, yet it can significantly enable you to get more work done by taking a break from work. Having fun triggers the brain in a way that enhances the capacity.

Takeaway: Set time out of your week for hobbies or events that you find interesting.

- Stimulate the Mind

Keep an activated but not overstressed mind. Mental struggles will give you energy, but too much can make you exhausted and frustrated. You can become tired and groggy without adequate difficulties, so try acquiring a new skill to activate your mind.

Takeaway: Ensure to push yourself with a unique adventure or objective every day.

- Meditate

Most individuals think that meditation is a perfect way to improve mental energy. A fundamental concept of meditation is just to be mind and breath mindful, and it has been proven to have a range of health values that may help improve your energy levels.

The intention is not to worry about the future or the past but to be conscious when meditating. I consider meditation as a time to openly let my imaginations run and take note of my feelings, ideas, and body.

Takeaway: Search for a meditation class next to you.

- Try New Stuff

Your mind will go into "auto-pilot" if you hold too closely to the same schedule. Mental stimulation is important for boosting energy, as described earlier.

Try to break the cycle and try something new. To offer yourself a new outlook, go on a fun ride. Go to a library and select a random book from a category you usually don't read.

Takeaway: Pick a task that you do regularly and change it in some way.

- Practice Minimalism

In personal life, learn to say "no" and remove waste. Trash whatever you don't need. There is more space for the stuff you want whenever you have fewer things in your life.

- Concentrate on what you can manage.

Stoics believe in concentrating on what is under our power. Our tranquility can be interrupted by needing or hoping for items that are not in our reach, and thinking about or wishing for something we don't have an effect on can lead to anxiety.

Takeaway: List what you are thinking or hoping for and separate what is under your power from what is not.

- Do what you are passionate about

Taking part in things that you're enthusiastic about, socially and professionally, tends to bring more satisfaction. It can be frustrating to spend time on things that you do not enjoy.

Takeaway: What do you enjoy doing? How can you organize your work or lifestyle to maximize energy so you can do more of it?

- Take responsibility For your feelings

Feelings have a strong influence on the levels of energy. You'll have less motivation if you're feeling sad or ashamed. You'll have more energy if you're feeling proud or optimistic.

You can become less reliant on external affirmation or situations to affect energy levels by accepting responsibility for your feelings.

- Be Present

Looking into the past or future negatively may cause anxiety. Consider the situation in which you are and take the best possible action. It will only create stress if you hope you were in a better position or hope you had done anything differently in the past.

Wrap Up Message

Each of the strategies above can be integrated into your everyday routine to boost your mental energy. Identify what causes you to lack energy, and attempt some of the above to improve your energy level and minimize exhaustion without the energy drink or additional cup of coffee, besides having a good night's sleep, exercise, and eating well.

Chapter 6: PREVENT PROCRASTINATION

How Procrastination Operates

The first question is the simplest one to address, so we're not going to spend a lot of time on it. Procrastination is the practice of stopping or putting off anything that ought to be done. In procrastination, the main element is that the hesitation is unreasonable. We know it isn't healthy to postpone a particular mission, but we do it nonetheless.

The reason we do it is the tougher question to answer. Why are we holding off doing something that would be to our greatest advantage?

When it's certainly beneficial to us, why do we put off going to the gym? Why do we postpone learning when it's what we need to do? Why do we delay the taxes before we get several notices and have to pay a fine?

(Hint: This is because there is a part of us that doesn't like to do this stuff.)

When Feelings Get in the Way

Procrastination has a lot to do with our feelings. Think of the last time you postponed anything you felt was important to get accomplished. Did you find any of the below feelings that went through your head?

"I'm not currently feeling like it."

"Maybe tomorrow I'll feel more like doing it."

"I don't wish to do this right now."

"I'm simply not in the right frame of mind."

This reluctance stems from the monkey's urge to resist whatever feels bad and prevent undesirable feelings. The activities you procrastinate in often inspire adverse feelings—frustration, fear, panic, boredom, and irritation. The monkey turns up each time you encounter bad feelings, urging you to alleviate such feelings.

And what is the convenient way to prevent such feelings? Simply put off the assignment, a feeling rolling through your mind. Phew, what a great relief! You feel great now that you are not dealing with that daunting task. But how long? This satisfaction, as I'm confident that you understand, is typically for a short time.

Any initial practice of procrastination will come back to haunt you pretty soon.

Are Procrastinators Simply Lazy?

I have been the type of guy who has boasted about my procrastination for much of my life. For instance, around three weeks before exams, I would never devote time to study at college. I couldn't stop procrastinating. But that isn't what I said to my colleagues. The explanation that I gave them, however, was that I really didn't care. I presented myself as a friendly kid who simply didn't give a fuck regarding anything.

This kind of conduct renders people believe that procrastinators are only lazy and reckless when the reverse is the case in reality: procrastinators care far too much. Procrastinators, whether or not they are conscious of it, are continually worried.

What they're doing is not good enough.

People will "discover the reality" about them.

People will discover that they are not as knowledgeable as they think.

They could get mocked

They are deficient and so on

Procrastination typically emerges from some panic: fear of failure, fear of accomplishment, fear of the unknown, fear of decision, fear of reprisal.

It's much simpler to procrastinate than to put in the effort and write a book and risk not being liked by people. It is much simpler to procrastinate than to launch a company and face failure.

Procrastinators appear to think a lot, whatever the actual trends are. When facing those tasks, they feel more bad feelings than "normal" individuals. Consequently, they also require more energy and greater ability for emotion control than average individuals do.

Sadly, many procrastinators never gain any skills in self-determination or emotion control. Procrastination is the single coping strategy many of us build.

Procrastination becomes a pattern after applying this technique for a while. And behaviors are difficult to break.

So, many procrastinators aren't reckless or lazy. They have profound emotional problems that need high determination and a well-built ability to control emotions, two things that are not available to the average procrastinator.

Despite these challenges, we will learn how to behave and get things done.

This is the key approach that worked for me, and I'm sure it's going to work for you, irrespective of your field or the nature of the procrastination challenges you're going through.

Steps Used to Combat Procrastination

- Awareness

Awareness is the very first move in any significant and lasting improvement. The change will be based on good fortune or incidental, without awareness. Reflect on this: how will you manage to fix it when you're not aware of what exactly is going wrong with your life? If you don't understand how, where, when, and why you procrastinate, how will you prevent it from happening?

You probably won't be reading this section of the book without awareness.

Besides, you wouldn't even be conscious that you're a procrastinator, and you would not be mindful that procrastination is a massive concern that you ought to be focused on for improvement.

Therefore, bravo to you. Unlike many of your other procrastinators, that have no idea what is happening in their lives, you have already learned that this is a part of yourself that you have to work on.

More so, by buying and studying this book, you have taken steps to fix this problem. And who knows what other things you've even tried?

The tragic fact is that 99% of individuals out there would never even know that they are procrastinating, let alone taking the measures required to solve it. You're simply ahead in the race. And when you continue reading and begin applying the techniques in this chapter, the effect of procrastination on your life will slowly but greatly be rid of.

You'll increase your productivity along the way and be a stronger, happier, and more efficient individual.

We have to be mindful of what's happening. Only then are we given the ability to alter anything.

- Build Your Unconscious Mind to Automatically Procrastinate Less

Wouldn't it be awesome if, in the long run, you were able to build yourself to behave in whatever way you like?

Maybe you could simply write a code for actions and afterward find yourself executing the code immediately?

If you were able to plan today, how will you act tomorrow?

- Implementation Intention

Well, great news, with the application of implementation intentions, you can do just that. Implementation intentions are if-then plans that reflect the way you will behave in a particular future scenario. They're going to look like this:

"If _____ happens, then i will do _____."

"I'll jump out of bed quickly as soon as I wake up." "If I'm done eating the food, then I'll clean all the plates immediately and tidy up the kitchen."

You are now choosing how you will behave in the future. This helps you to make judgments from a place of peace and logic. You might ask yourself, "What would be the greatest way to go about things if this or that happened?" What else would I want to try if so and so did happen? After completing XYZ, what else would I like doing? "

Intentions for implementation can appear too simple to be successful. However, they are one of the most practiced and tested modern psychology techniques to influence people's actions significantly.

Why do Intentions for Implementation Perform so Well?

What develops in our minds as we are shaping these implementation intentions is interesting. First, a connection between the cue and the behavior desired is established. If you were to go to the gym center after returning home from the workplace, you would establish the following plan: "I'll go to the gym center as soon as I return home from the workplace." In this scenario, the cue "returning home from work" would be correlated with the behavior "heading to the gym center."

Next, the cue gets strongly triggered in your brain. This implies that the cue is simply dying to get noticed. It's sort of like a schoolchild putting his hand up in enthusiasm and seeking to have the teacher's attention.

Your brain is now continuously searching the environment in quest of the cue without any concerted effort or consciousness of your own (e.g., "returning home from work").

Set Certain Intentions For Implementation

Take a couple of minutes to think about your patterns of procrastination.

About what activities do you prefer to procrastinate? When are you most vulnerable to procrastination? What events would you like to participate in more frequently? What new habits do you want to create?

When you reflect on procrastination in your personal life, you will find plenty of options for using the implementation intentions.

Note down several if-then strategies for your best concepts and repeat them a few times out loud or in your mind.

And don't worry about keeping the particular if-then equation in your strategies. You're ready to party it as long as you're connecting a cue to the desired action.

Chapter 7: BOOST YOUR PRODUCTIVITY

Strategies to Boost Your Productivity at Work

There are several hours in the day, and therefore it is important to make the most out of your time. There are broadly two ways to boost your overall productivity within the hours of the day—either putting in more hours or working more intelligently. I'm not going to speak for you, but the latter one I prefer.

It's not rocket science to be more efficient at work, but it involves being more conscious about handling your time, irrespective of your field and profession. This chapter will present you with easy but productive strategies to boost your work productivity.

- Monitor and restrict how much time you spend on activities.

You may assume you're particularly great at calculating how much time you spend on different activities. Nevertheless, certain studies show that only about 17 percent of individuals can correctly measure the passing of time. A device such as Rescue Time will help by letting you know precisely how much time you spend on everyday activities, including social media, policy formulation session email, training, business meeting, and apps.

- Consider taking breaks frequently.

It seems counterproductive, but it can potentially help boost focus by taking planned breaks. Many studies have revealed that it allows you to maintain a sustained level of productivity by taking brief breaks during long practice sessions, gyming activities, business conferences, etc.; working on a task for long hours without breaks results in a gradual decrease in productivity.

- Develop deliberate deadlines.

While we generally assume stress as a negative thing, a reasonable amount of deliberate stress can help us concentrate and achieve our goals. Start setting yourself a deadline for indefinite tasks or jobs, and then adhere to it. Anytime you check the clock, you can be shocked to learn just how concentrated and efficient you can be.

- Employ the "two-minute rule."

To make the most of the tiny chunks of time at your disposal at work, entrepreneur Steve Olenski suggests enforcing the "two-minute rule." The principle is this: If you see a job or activity that you believe can be completed in two minutes or less, do it instantly. According to Olenski, it simply consumes less time to complete the task straight away than trying to come back to it later. This is equally true for any profession where there are usually well-defined activities to be undertaken.

- Say no to meetings.

Meetings are one of the greatest time-sucks around, but still, we manage to book them unquestionably, hold them, and moan about them eventually. According to Atlassian, in unproductive meetings, the average businessman consumes around 31 hours per month. Before scheduling your next meeting, consider asking yourself if you can achieve the same objectives or jobs through email, smartphone, or web-based meeting (that could be overtly more productive).

- Hold a standing meeting.

Suppose you need to have a meeting. In that case, there's a certain indication that standing meetings (they're simply what they seem like—everybody stands) may lead to greater group arousal, reduced territoriality, and enhanced group productivity. This is especially necessary for the army and certain other forces, where the members' complete alertness is needed.

- Stop Multitasking.

Although we prefer to think of the ability to multitask as a significant ability to maximize productivity, the reverse can be true. Research has found that trying to accomplish numerous tasks simultaneously may lead to a loss of time and productivity. Instead, before moving on to the next task, develop a habit of sticking to a single assignment.

- Using your time to your advantage.

This applies to any unforeseen "bonus" time that writer Miranda Marquit indicates you can find on your hands. Use the time to hammer out those addresses, visit the gym, go o a short training, build your regular to-do list, or try some strategizing for your business rather than Candy-Crushing or Facebooking.

- Give up on the fantasy of perfection.

For business people, it is normal to get caught up in trying to perfect a task—the fact is that nothing is ever perfect. Instead of wasting so much time pursuing this fantasy, hammer your assignment out to the best possible standard and move on. It is easier to finish the assignment and get it off your plate; you can simply come back and change or strengthen it later if need be.

- Take breaks from exercise.

According to a study in the Occupational and Environmental Medicine journal, utilizing work hours to exercise can boost productivity. Build in a set period over the week to take a stroll or go to the gym, if necessary. It might be simply what's required to clear your mind and get your attention back and get your blood flowing.

- Be constructive rather than reactive.

Enabling incoming calls and messages to decide how you spend your day would imply you do a better job of putting out fires by —but that could be all you get done. Take some time to reply to emails, though don't let them decide how your day will look like. Develop a plan of work at the beginning of every day, and then try your best to adhere to it."

- Switch the notifications off.

No one can be assumed to resist the charm of notification via email, voicemail, or message. Switch off your alerts throughout work time, and instead create time to go over your email and texts. All this is indicative of being constructive instead of reactive.

- Working at intervals of 90 minutes.

Florida State University studies have identified that elite professionals (athletes, politicians, singers, etc.) working at intervals of not greater than 90 minutes are more effective than those working 90 minutes or more. They equally discovered that experts with top performance appear to work not more than 4.5 hours a day. Appear s great to me!

- Give yourself a pretty thing to glance at.

This might sound impossible, but certain studies show that equipping an office or working space with aesthetically appealing components like plants—can improve productivity by up to 25%. Beautify your workplace or training room with frames, candles, roses, or something else that leaves a smile on your face.

Morning Routine and Productivity

The advantages that you can discover when you integrate a morning routine into your everyday life will be special to you. During the day, specific individuals feel they're more efficient. Others find that they feel more secure and attentive. Others are also shocked to discover that they feel more motivated, optimistic, and concentrated when carrying out a purposeful morning routine.

After a week or two, many individuals find that the idea of waking up doesn't overwhelm them anymore. In reality, since they realize their routines will help them have a good day, they look forward to waking up early.

You will encounter advantages that will change your life, literally.

- It will offer your day a structure

Every morning, adopting a conscious and carefully crafted routine will give your day a better structure. The repetition of your desired tasks will make your morning and the rest of your day more reliable. This, in essence, will assist you in taking on tasks of greater effectiveness.

- You'll feel better energy

Several morning activities can significantly improve your productivity. And, above all, some of them can help make sure that your energy levels don't drop in the middle of the morning.

For instance, you'll feel refreshed by doing some workouts, going for a quick walk, and eating a high-protein breakfast. Many individuals think that the secret is to practice yoga, meditate, and take a cold shower.

- You'll be less vulnerable to decision fatigue

The more you make choices, the poorer the standard of those decisions. This result is called decision fatigue. You get less capable of managing your emotions and making reasonable decisions as this form of fatigue sets in.

The amount of decisions you make in the morning is reduced by a morning routine. The tasks you select become a routine, which avoids the difficult task of determining whether to do them.

Making fewer options in the morning helps you to retain your energy for the remainder of the day for decision.

- During the day, you'll be productive

From firsthand experience, you're acquainted with this outcome. You seem more in charge of your day whenever your morning begins well. This emotion is partially due to having a good mindset. Part of it is because of getting more willpower, feeling more energetic, and less tension. And part of that comes from having a good understanding of what you have to do all day long.

With a consistent morning routine, your brain is prepared to deal with the unavoidable everyday difficulties and obstacles which would otherwise disrupt your productivity.

Chapter 8: DECISION MAKING

Strategies Used In Intuitive Decision Making

We could apply intuition when we have no chance of building up a lot of experience. When confronted with unexpected problems, we still need to depend on intuition. We have no alternative. None of us begins as a master in selecting the right business deal, choosing the right alternative, going on the right mission, committing to a course, deciding who can be trusted in a team or evaluating your opponent's move. As we move along, we understand. Except in these situations, here is some guidance for making effective use of intuition in decision making.

- It is possible that the first choice you think of would be the best.

That's not a promise. Only an assumption backed up by proof from studies. So, if confronted with a tough decision, it is essential to note your original impulses. You need to think carefully about this choice. Perhaps you can neglect it. However, if you neglect it, you will lose out on some quick and free guidance from your inner self. But, if you simply can't select between different choices after reasoning about your decision, you can maybe just go with the first instinct.

- Employ analysis to help your instinct.

That implies being conscious of what your instincts are saying to you before using your intuition. Assess your first instinct by considering how your decision will be carried out and the things that could go wrong in a manner that draws on your experience. That's what soldiers and business people and other trained decision-makers do as they envision how a circumstance would play out in the here-and-now to determine their decisions. They don't evaluate choices out of context to see if they line up on a standard set of parameters. You're going to get detached from your instincts when you tear up the decision in that manner.

Put more focus into knowing the scenario than on worrying about what to do. You may ponder all day. However, your choice of action is not guaranteed to be quite successful when you don't realize what's going on. To understand the circumstances and the implications, you are better off using your time. Doing so renders it more possible for your instincts to contribute to surprising ideas.

- Don't mistake intuition with lust.

They are never the same. We all know ladies, for instance, that continue dating the wrong kind of guys, overlooking the red flags over and over again. What was going on with their intuition? Oh, nothing. These ladies understand their new lovers have the same issues as the previous ones. Their intuition is okay. They are dismissing these intuitions since stronger factors are involved. Their eventual suffering is a message to all of us on what can happen if our intuitions are disregarded.

Override your intuitions anytime they fool you. Bear in mind that intuitions are not faultless. It is important to check them out. Without thought, one risk of applying intuition is that we may get fixated. Even though we don't, we can assume we understand a circumstance, but instead, we make this problem even worse by neglecting all the contradictory evidence. Our brains are very great at hanging on to false convictions. Check if you are in the grasp of obsession to break free. For instance, consider asking yourself if there is some proof that might cause you to change your mind. If not, then you will get stuck. It's not simple to get unstuck, and our interpretation of events is often just too convincing. Try to create an alternative narrative, give yourself some space for cognitive thinking, and watch what unfolds.

- Just think ahead.

Intuition will help us think ahead of the curve by generating assumptions, bridging the gap, flagging contradictions, or informing us of complications. Using thorough consideration of circumstances, the universe is too complicated to plan. Instead, we need to depend on our intuition. However, we need to offer intuition an opportunity to depend upon it. For instance, it is not sufficient to just listen to a supervisor or senior officer's task and commit it to memory. The individuals who display the greatest capacity to plan consciously try to visualize how the task will be carried out. In their heads, they process it through, visualizing how the scenario would go down to see whether any intuitive warnings are received. Their attitude of engagement is unique from the passive attitude we experience every day. The next time you need to navigate anywhere unknown and are offered complicated guidance and a fuzzy route to follow, do more than just note each of the bends and the road's address to switch onto. Try to visualize how you're going to drive the road, get a picture of the path you're going to be headed, try to foresee where you may get stuck or confused, and request more specific risk mitigation instructions. This strategy meets the need to think ahead.

- Ambiguity brings enthusiasm to decision-making.

A foundational element of intuitive decision-making is ambiguity. When faced with confusion, so many individuals get irritated. They let confusion debilitate them or send them off on a wild goose chase for details that will come too late and will still not be enough to respond to all the questions. Reflect on this. Where would the problem be when we had great knowledge all the time? Intuition development allows us to handle ambiguity:

to embrace it as unavoidable, to recognize when to collect more details, and to feel when, amid the unaddressed questions, to move on. The lack of ambiguity ought to make us tense. It may suggest that we are oversimplifying, ignoring potentially significant facts. For instance, if we need to make a tough decision, we want everything to assemble. We like to fix all the loose ends by explaining that one of the alternatives truly dominates the rest and is superior in every respect. Our conscious mind is searching for continuity, which is why, before everything falls inline, we continue excruciating. We're excellent at describing away the loose ends.

Nevertheless, doing so would be an error since lapses are unavoidable. It's a red flag if something lines up too perfectly. You might be trying to deceive yourself when you do not have to consider any trade-offs in the process of choosing.

- Using the best approach for decision-making.

There is a moment to depend on intuition and a moment to examine all the variables going into a decision. Analytical decisions are typically foolish, as the method depends on random evaluations and possible inconsistencies, only if the key problems could be described in numbers. However, if the situations are complex and no one has a clear understanding of the entire situation, research makes more sense than intuitions. There is also a moment to admit that we are in the indifference zone and that we can not draw a conclusion preferring one alternative over the other, irrespective of how hard we try. When the benefits and drawbacks of your choices cancel each other out, the indifference zone exists. In as much as you have willpower and endurance, you may fight "in the zone," though you may as well toss a coin since you're not going to escape through evaluation or intuition.

- Try to consult the experts.

If we are in new fields, such as business investment planning, we can value experts' insights rather than our intuition. But who's an expert, though? If various people assert knowledge but offer you conflicting advice, you will need to figure out the imposter experts. The actual experts can: recognize small clues that you have not observed, use detailed thought patterns of how things function, and implement solutions that you have not considered. Real professionals love coming up with workarounds. Typically, experts think two or three levels beyond the rest of us. Since they are equally seeking to learn to be different, they are still mindful of their faults. When someone cannot recall a time when he or she previously made an error, be wary. When you trust an expert, tap into that individual's instincts by asking for details, past events, or how you think the present circumstance will play out.

Stay alert because of obstacles to intuition. Warning signs should go up If you experience any of these circumstances at an organization:

- Systems have been designed to reassure others that all they need to do is obey the protocols. Management is irritated when someone finds out weaknesses or contradictions in the "typical" way of doing things.
- A community in which individuals are deemed well educated can memorize the steps required to do their job.
- The knowledge of the key staff is not respected by management. Bosses want workers to follow directives without being provided the opportunity to explain them.
- Management is uncertainty intolerant and depends on large quantities of data gathering as a remedy for uncertainty. Systems allow everybody to handle by applying simple numerical objectives to make it transparent.
- Management is starting to search for ways to replace human expertise with computer technology.
- An indication that your own intuition won't be respected is either of these obstacles. But these situations can be opportunities as well. You should expect the company to run into trouble (predictably) and plan to apply your intuitions to help the division recover.

Chapter 9: ELIMINATE NEGATIVE THINKING

Reformulate All Negative Thinking

Whether you assume that you can, or you believe that you can't, either way, you are right!" Henry Ford. For survival and for thriving in a modern age, our thought processes are vital. Creative thinking offers us the opportunity to rapidly and efficiently solve problems. Creative thinking helps us to derive insights and associations that are unique, dynamic, and comprehensive. But it is the negative, uninvited thought that clogs up our minds and sometimes consumes our passion for life.

"According to Australian expert Dr. Russ Harris, author of The Happiness Trap: How to Stop Struggling and Start Living, "Therefore, evolution has structured our minds so that we are configured that way to struggle psychologically: to assess, analyze, and criticize ourselves, to concentrate on the things we lack, to get unhappy with what we possess easily, and to envision all kinds of terrifying scenarios. No doubt human beings find it difficult to be happy! "

Most individuals spend their whole lives plagued by their negative feelings. They assume that they have no power over what ideas exist in their minds, or much worse. They acknowledge the "voices" in their minds warning them that the world will end. While the stigma of negativity is true, the attempts towards a shift and self-awareness are not impervious. While it can feel normal to encourage your head to drift into fear and depression, you have strengthened negative thinking by not questioning it and embracing your feelings as your identity. But by developing the reformulating habit, you can understand this inclination and alter it.

The first step is to recognize and disrupt your thinking patterns before they get out of hand. Here are six techniques you can use to smash the pattern and start taming your mind during your day. It takes only a couple of minutes to implement every one of these tactics.

- Be Watchful

Begin by being conscious of your thinking. Detach yourself from your emotions and simply watch what is happening in your head. The secret here is to do this in an objective way in which you judge no individual opinion. Be mindful of yourself as a distant observer to your ideas. It is possible to do this exercise occasionally over the day or during meditation practice. The ideas and feelings they foster are disempowered by witnessing your thoughts instead of attaching to them.

- Alter your Thought

Another means to isolate yourself from your worries is by psychologically accepting that they are nothing but emotions and not your reality. For instance, if you feel, "I'm not going to have all of these done," alter the psychological dialog to "I'm thinking I'm not going to get all of these done." This confirms the fact that you are not your feelings.

- Say No

Whenever you find yourself in a psychological loop or concern, just say, "No!" out loud (verbalizing enhances the disruption), and then imagine a hard rock wall crashing down right in front of your uncontrolled thoughts.

- Apply the rubber band Strategy

Attach a rubber band around your hand. Anytime you see it, hold and notice your thoughts. Place the rubber band on the second wrist or pop it softly on your wrist when you are lost in negative thought. This physical action disrupts the flow of negative thinking.

- Understand the Causes

Sometimes, an individual, circumstance, or physical condition causes excessive thinking and negativity. Pay close attention to the usual fears and problems you are brooding over. Is there something that arises in your mind that triggers them? If so, note down the causes so that anytime they arise, you're conscious of them. This knowledge will enable you to prevent negative thoughts from consuming you.

- Distract Yourself

End the cycle by using distractions. Try something that's going to fill your head so that the negative thoughts have no space. Indulge yourself in an activity that requires intellectual capacity and attention.

- Acknowledge the facts about anxiety

Acknowledge that anxiety is always abstract. When you take action, you will do better than when you do not do anything and allow the negative thoughts to consume you.

I recently read about 20-year old research stating that 85 percent of the things individuals fear never exist and that their answer is generally much better than they assume to the other 10 percent.

- Use plenty of affirmations

Read some of Napoleon Hill's works, and you'll realize he had an immense appreciation for affirmations. And from my opinion and knowledge, when a man that interviewed a few of his age's richest men suggests that affirmations are great, then they're likely perfect.

Affirmations help as they offer the brain something to concentrate on rather than flooding it with unwanted negative thoughts. You really should know that even if you say "I'm wealthy," a million times a day would not make you a rich man automatically. Emphasizing any affirmation over and over practically forces you to go out of your comfort zone and take action.

I apply affirmations a lot, and I stand by them. I build one affirmation for every one of my targets each month, and I simply repeat it again and again in leisure, office, or training sessions. Whenever I feel lazy or frustrated, I still apply these affirmations, and I typically get back to work with enthusiasm and perseverance inside minutes.

- Write down your thoughts in a diary

Thoughts come and go so easily that you do not remember what caused you to feel unpleasant about something. The remedy?

Note down the things that trouble you. This is called journaling or creative writing by professionals and is a perfect way to handle negativity. One research by the University of Michigan showed that students appear to do much better when they report their problems before a difficult test.

Another report on 1,300 returning U.S. veterans discovered that four weekly periods of writing things down for five consecutive weeks were perfect for enabling them to deal with post-war anxiety.

Using the popular techniques of Cognitive Behavior Therapy to evaluate your unhealthy negative thoughts is another idea that could make writing things down much more successful. Such trends are:

Everything-or-nothing

Catastrophising

Discounting the positive result:

Thinking about something is real because you believe it's true (Aka. Emotional reasoning)

Labeling stuff or yourself (Ex: I am a loser)

Overgeneralisation (Ex: Everybody hates me)

Personalization: Believing others are acting adversely because of you

Applying imperatives: by using a lot of should and must, binding yourself with several laws

- Always foresee winning

Many individuals don't think it's beneficial as they're afraid of getting upset. The reality, nevertheless, is that planning to win improves your chances of winning much more than anticipating failure.

I was going through Roland Lazenby's biography of Michael Jordan, and his winning theory was so straightforward but mind-changing. Jordan felt that he had to anticipate each shot to hit the ring to gather most of his shots.

He realized that no side wins each match and no player scores every shot, but the individuals who regularly win are people who are really in it to win it, the Jordans of life. Every single time around. When you start to think this manner, you'll feel incredibly productive, and everything you do, you'll become a Jordan.

- Get adequate sleep

I know this might appear off-point. However, the reality is, most individuals underestimate adequate sleep. I listened to LeBron James talk regarding his schedule with Tim Ferris, and he said more than once that it's just about sufficient sleep and healthy rest.

Lack of sleep will rub off on your brain and attitude (not to mention your immune system, sex drive, and blood pressure). Therefore, it could be only a product of your poor sleep patterns to think negatively.

Chapter 10: SOLID SELF-CONFIDENCE

The Fundamentals of Self-Confidence

Have you ever said to yourself, what if I become more confident? Are you willing to attempt some fun things, however, lose your courage after that? Do you postpone attending the gym, going to a team meeting, starting up your new business, going for daily training, or communicating your true feelings to that unique person in your life?

Have you hesitated to respond to such questions? Or was your instant response a YES? Irrespective of the circumstance, you lack the courage to take the step.

To be honest with you, many individuals struggle to grasp the true meaning of the word confidence. And that is the reason they're not feeling the confidence that can massively change their lives.

Building Confidence, The Four Stage Strategy

You can't take negative thinking lightly because it can simply and rapidly escalate out of hand and then harm your confidence without allowing you the opportunity to work for its enhancement. You require special techniques to monitor, disrupt, or avoid those thoughts and override them with more beneficial, constructive ones.

The technique we will address in this chapter is called The Four Stage Strategy. This simple but powerful approach helps you to recognize thinking patterns that are discouraging. You will stop them from being a regular aspect of your values and views until you become conscious of these feelings. You can learn this technique quickly and apply it and make it super easy.

You will build full self-confidence with this efficient technique and change your life completely for good.

To explore the four steps that make up this method, read on:

- Exercise Mindfulness

We say, by mindfulness, that you pay careful attention to anything you think and feel. Be careful of the manner you react to individuals and various circumstances. Your brain can better perceive and observe things more accurately as you get more responsive to these factors. Then you are less liable to make poor decisions or irrational ones. To be honest, your perception of yourself and the things around you is strengthened by mindfulness. It is the first step that you can undertake towards the development of tremendous self-confidence.

- Avoid Negative Thinking

Human beings do not behave like machines. It is possible to determine how to think, though a little complicated actively.

You have to begin adjusting your thought habits instantly if you want to develop your confidence.

Anytime you discover yourself developing negative feelings, stop yourself and ask, "Am I once more thinking negatively?" Am I a killjoy? Why am I finding it so difficult to think positively? Is my dialog packed with doom and gloom frequently?"

These questions, when answered honestly, will help you become conscious of your true nature. At this point, stop yourself and make a deliberate effort to avoid thinking negatively.

- Replace negative thoughts with a positive one

"If the responses to all the questions described in step 2 above are yes, consider asking yourself, "What have I achieved so far with my negative thinking? If I had more positive feelings, how confident will I be? Find out and note down a minimum of 5 differences that will render your life a positive thought template.

Try to manage and handle your emotions to refer to yourself in a stimulating and constructive way in all circumstances. Yes, some preparation might be needed, but it's certainly possible. Try using expressions like "I do," "I want," "I can," and "I am" that begin with positive words.

- Proceed until it becomes your norm

Once you can recognize, disrupt and substitute your negative feelings with positive ones, make a pledge to yourself that you would never use limiting words such as "I can't," "I'm not sure," or "I'm incapable" from this moment on. Ensure you don't ever let yourself down. Reassure yourself that everything is attainable; working hard is all you require.

"YES" is among the most powerful statements you can make. Say it always, vigorously. Anytime you have a new chance, remind yourself that you can make it all happen. Embrace any challenge or issue and put the best effort into making it work.

The Fundamentals of Unrelenting Self-Confidence

You have now entered the point where you can work on your confidence development plan after knowing the foundations of confidence, the indications of tremendous confidence, the triggers of a lack of confidence, and figuring out how internal emotions can be managed and adjusted.

So how will you be able to build this acute sense of stable self-confidence based on a profound appreciation of fact? The fact is that no easy fix is available. Nevertheless, if you have the courage and concentrate on pulling through, it will likely acquire massive confidence. Another incredible thing you have to realize is the methods you use to develop self-confidence can equally help you attain success. Self-confidence comes, after all, from actual accomplishments. And nobody has the authority to take this away from you.

So read on and discover your approach to developing great self-confidence.

Step 1: Get Ready For the Journey

The first and most critical step in building self-confidence is to brace yourself for the journey ahead. Note down your present state in this step, decide what you like to accomplish, evaluate your attitude, and make a promise to finish the journey irrespective of how tough.

Let us take a quick look at all of these steps.

Define Your Present Circumstance

Think of your life, the stuff you care about, and the things you like to do in the future. A significant aspect of this journey is to identify your objectives. This is where true confidence originates from—using the strategic planning process to make objectives realistic and then evaluate those goals' effective achievement.

Predict Your Future Self

Assume that your future self has infinite self-confidence, as opposed to your present self. Try to imagine how you think, communicate, stand, run, act, and do everything. Observe that.

Take a look at yourself. Sense what occurs when you are projecting solid confidence.

This training aspect is to make a firm commitment to yourself that you will finish the journey and do what you can to obtain absolute confidence.

Step 2: Set Out for the Journey

This is the stage in which you are starting to work towards your target. Start with simple, tiny accomplishments and proceed with your journey on the road to success.

Fix Previous Errors

When you've done something that is not right, revert to the past. You could not have made the proper effort, or you have done something that has just taken success away from you. Revert to the moment you strayed from your course of achievement, and substitute your dream outcome with the original ending. You're going to see how things seem and feel different. You'll discover yourself going around the world more confidently because your past has changed.

Defining and Scheduling Your Targets

Start with the tiny, basic objectives you have defined in the preceding step. Develop a habit of establishing your targets, meeting them, and enjoying them. At this point, refrain from making impossible targets, as this will make it hard for you to progress. And then pile up the wins.

- Phase III: Speed Up Towards Progress

You can see your confidence growing at this point. Now you can push yourself. Set bigger, more complicated goals. Broaden your obligations. Enhance your abilities.

Reach your Confidence Level

And this is where you find your confident new self. You can try things better at this point, consider new tasks, and connect with nearly everyone. In your posture, style, movements, and attitude, you and others will find a positive distinction. Every part of your character, after all, now reflects limitless confidence.

Chapter 11: REPROGRAM YOUR MIND

How to Reprogram Your Subconscious Mind

Are you enjoying the life that you always wished to live? Or did you settle for less?

Many of us have a fuzzy perception of what we believe we deserve. We also get disappointed and angry whenever life veers away from the course that we have secretly planned for. Why is this occurring? "We wonder. This frustration can be strong; it can motivate us to make a change.

However, discontent is a two-sided coin. Too many of us eventually turn our resentment and anger toward ourselves, jeopardizing any future success. We begin to think that we deserve better, and for a few days, we can push a little more complicated. Still, instead of taking action and working for long-term change, we slip right back to where we think we belong in our jobs, our finances, our businesses, our wellness, our overall feeling of well-being.

What if you took back your mind's active power and focused your energy on making your life better? What if your mind is reprogrammed to build a life that gives you happiness, excitement, and passion?

Your mind is the secret to happiness, and you can understand the way your subconscious mind can be reprogrammed. To devote and to resolve, it's necessary to consider if you wish to enjoy the life you desire. In life, it's not the things we can do that bring a difference. It's what we're going to do. And there is no reasonable opportunity right now to wield back your mind's power and focus your attention on something great.

Do you wish to master the way to reprogram your subconscious mind for excellence? Below are the steps that you must take to get you underway.

- **Step 1: Decide**

The very first step you have to take is to acquire a total understanding of what you desire. Master how to avoid excessive thinking and concentrate on your objectives. What is your intended result? What do you think discovering an incredible life will seem like? Clarity is essential. The more thinking you put into this, the more information you put out, the greater and more effective your goal will get. It generates a subconscious mind map, providing the mind with the required resources to transform the vision into reality.

Would you like to learn the way your subconscious mind may be reprogrammed? Try an argument with your colleague. We sometimes lose sight of the dispute itself while in a verbal argument with a colleague or business partner and concentrate on being heard, on making the final word, on prevailing. You quit watching your language and being polite with your wife and start to treat them as an enemy. This is a fast way for the conflict to turn into something even worse. Resist this urge instead, and think, "Why am I arguing in the first place?" You are trying to fight; you are simply disagreeing with something and need a resolution. You lose sight of the real issue when you are overwhelmed by winning. When you realize that, you can turn your attention back to addressing the original problem, reprogramming your mind efficiently to use its energy and delivering the result at that point.

Reprogramming the mind begins with determining and reflecting on what you desire in the present and future. Offer your mind guidance. Energy flows where concentration goes. In your company and in your professional life, what is it you desire physically, economically, mentally, and psychologically? Decide that you are not ready to settle down and that right now, you are not ready to continue with the way you live. Focus your attention on the things you want and launch your mind reprogramming.

- **Step 2: Commit**

The next step in mind reprogramming is to commit once you determine the things you want. Get rid of anxiety and self-doubt in your brain. How will you achieve that? By making a decision, committing to it, and letting it propel you.

One of the main pitfalls which prevent individuals from taking action is fear. Fear of acceptance, fear of loss, success, misery, the unexpected. We all have our fears. That fear will stay precisely where it is, restricting your way if you don't do anything. You're not going to move, and you're still going to live in fear. You may not be doing any worse, but you're not going to do better either. But right in the subconscious mind, the fear will always be there, driving you further from your objectives. The failure to act offers time for the negativity to infiltrate your feelings: "It's a great idea I haven't tried." When enabled to propagate into your subconsciousness, this anxiety-based negativity will percolate into all you feel about yourself and everything you do. I would never have done it.

Facing it immediately is the right way to handle fear and reprogram your subconscious. You have to look it straight in the eye and start taking steps despite it. Do you fear failure? Think of it this way: Failure is a means to learn. You'll know exactly what has not worked if you try something and fail. Once you attempt again, you'll have the ability to take a more trained, knowledgeable approach. It's great for you than where you were before.

Reprogramming your mind involves ending negative talk like "I can't." Reflect on it in a similar way you would build muscle at the gym. It will appear complicated initially and maybe even taxing. However, when you begin small and attempt again and again each time, you can get better rapidly. And sooner somewhat later, it will become an effortless habit.

Commit to yourself. Commit yourself to combat negativity. Commit to a decent life. You will drive yourself to the next stage and require more of yourself than any other person will ever demand once you commit entirely, cutting off all other possibilities. And that is the real strength of programming the minds.

- **Step 3: Resolve**

Take an inventory of your condition after you have agreed on your course and committed entirely. What are you earning from your present actions? Guide your mind towards analyzing what works and what doesn't. Make the changes. Resolve is about seeking answers to everything that might come your way.

Adaptability is a vital aspect of finding determination and successfully reprogramming the mind. You will lose out on prospects and alternate paths that could translate to amazing advantages. Tunnel vision sets restrictions on you. Know, you are never 100 percent in charge. Reflect on this: has your life ever gone as planned? Maybe not. The route that you follow is not a straight line. And that's the reason it is important to stay adaptive all along the way, growing from failures, accepting disappointment, and using negativity as a motivating force for change. You are heading in the right direction as long as you are making headway.

You gain the opportunity to adjust your attitude to issues when needed as you reprogram your mind to concentrate on solving them. Not all barriers, challenges, or situations are the same; each presents its unique challenges, and you can face such challenges head-on. Ultimate strength emerges from inside, and reprogramming your mind conditions you for progress. Frustration becomes a blessing since it indicates you are on the brink of success. Failure becomes an experience to advise you in the future about how to do better. Every obstacle becomes a chance for you to adjust and find a new innovative approach. That is the strength of your mind's dedication to resolving.

Useful Tips to Reprogram the Mind

- Embrace Empowering Beliefs

Restricting beliefs hold people back from the things they want in life. They can be focused on previous outcomes, adverse events that they have witnessed, or a faulty view of their future. They will substitute them with empowering beliefs to thrive when they approach these convictions and question their accuracy. What does it look like? "It could be substituting "My father was not a good athlete. Therefore, it's in my genetic material it's not to win a gold medal" with "I deserve a gold medal in a competitive tournament." You change the world if you change your mindset.

- Embrace The Beauty of Uncertainty

We are never in charge of life; our acts and responses are the sole things we can control. We take back our ability to influence our life and reprogram our minds when we accept this idea. Let go of the urge for assurance and enjoy the beauty of uncertainty. We can let go and enjoy the journey when we concentrate on selecting trust, sharing without caring about what we get in exchange, and living actively.

- Concentrate On Gratitude

You shed light on the positive If you pick gratitude and respect over resentment and fear. To focus more on the things you have and less on what you don't reprograms your mind. When you no longer regard them with skepticism, it also helps you be informed about your life. You should accept change and let it in, knowing that life rarely remains the same.

- Monitor The Environment

You need to restrict toxic stimuli in your life when reprogramming your mind for progress. Your subconscious mind is actively consuming external sources of knowledge and using the data to create perceptions that affect the way you think and act. Without you consciously realizing it, negativity from daily news, negative people, and business competitors can greatly influence your subconsciousness.

Note that proximity is a force as you focus on the way to reprogram your mind. Associate yourself with positive, helpful friends. Check for articles, podcasts, and programs that encourage you and lifts you up. You will learn with time that your subconscious mind is more optimistic and motivating and that negative emotions have decreased considerably.

- Visualize

What does your dream day seem like? Where do you want to go about your massive presentation at work? How do you like the first tournament to go, exactly? How will your first extradition mission going to be? Choose something you are genuinely committed to making a possibility and devote 10-15 minutes of your time visualizing it every day as though it had already occurred.

Chapter 12: DEVELOP EVERLASTING SELF-ESTEEM

Enhancing Self-Esteem

Self-esteem is the way you feel about yourself or the perception you develop about yourself. Everybody has moments where they feel a little vulnerable or find it difficult to trust themselves. Nevertheless, this may result in complications when this becomes a long-term condition, like mental health problems such as depression or anxiety. An indication of such issues may also be some of the signs of poor self-esteem.

Self-esteem is always the product of experiences over a lifetime, specifically what occurred to us as kids. At any age, nevertheless, it is likely to increase our self-esteem. This chapter provides more self-esteem details and some strategies that you can follow to enhance it.

Understanding Self-Esteem

Certain individuals think of self-esteem as their internal voice (or self-dialogue), informing them whether they are good enough to do or accomplish anything.

Typically, self-esteem is about the way we value ourselves and our opinions of the person we are and the things we are capable of.

Self-esteem is not connected with your ability. Self-esteem is also not correlated with either your ability or the impressions people have about you. It is possible for an individual who is excellent at something to have low self-esteem. In comparison, somebody who is struggling with a specific task may usually have high self-esteem. Typically, individuals with high self-esteem feel better about themselves and their life. It allows them much more flexibility, and they are better able to deal with life's adversities.

Nevertheless, those who have low self-esteem are also even more skeptical of themselves. They find it more difficult to come back from struggles and losses. This can drive them to avoid complicated circumstances. However, it may potentially further lower their self-esteem since they feel somewhat worse about themselves as a result.

So, the absence of self-esteem will impact the way individuals act, not to say what they accomplish in their lives.

Strategies Used in Enhancing Self-Esteem

There is a range of strategies through which you can increase your self-esteem.

- Identifying and challenging your negative thoughts

The first step is to recognize your negative thought and then challenge them. Note the feelings you have about yourself. You can discover yourself saying, for instance, 'I'm not smart enough to achieve that or 'I have no peers.' Look for proof that disputes those claims once you do. To reassure yourself that your negative thoughts about yourself are not valid, note down both claims and facts and continue looking back at them.

- Recognize the positive things about yourself

It's equally a great idea to note down positive things about yourself, like being great at a sport, business, fighting, or something that individuals have mentioned about you that is pleasant. Reflect on such things when you begin to feel low, and reassure yourself that there are many positives in you.

Good self-talk, in particular, is a significant aspect of raising your self-esteem.

If you hear yourself thinking things like 'I'm not good enough at the last training' or 'I'm a loser, I made the mess of my last business negotiation' you can start turning things around by saying 'I can beat this' and ' I can get more confident by seeing myself more optimistically.'

To begin with, you may discover yourself slipping back on old bad habits, but you will start to feel more optimistic and develop your self-esteem with daily effort.

- Constructing positive relationships and avoiding negative ones

You will discover that some individuals and some relationships cause you to feel better than others. Try to stop them if there are individuals who cause you to feel bad about yourself. Develop relationships with individuals that make you feel positive about yourself and prevent relationships that weigh you down.

- Give Yourself a Break

You don't need to be flawless each hour of the day. Every time, you need not have to feel great about yourself. Self-esteem differs from circumstance to circumstance, from week to week, and from minute to minute. With friends and coworkers, certain individuals feel comfortable and optimistic but nervous and awkward with outsiders. Some may feel absolutely in charge of themselves at work, yet suffer socially (or vice versa).

Offer yourself a break. We all have moments when we feel a little discouraged or find it more difficult to retain our self-confidence. The trick is to not be too tough on ourselves. Be compassionate and not too mean to ourselves. Do not criticize yourself against others, as this will strengthen your negative feelings and equally give other people a (probably false) negative impression towards you.

You may help improve your self-esteem by offering yourself a reward anytime you can do something tough or simply to survive a terrible day.

- Get more assertive and learn to say no

It is also difficult for individuals with poor self-esteem to speak up for themselves or say no to certain things. This suggests that they may get overwhelmed at home, work, or the business place since they do not want to deny someone anything. Nevertheless, this can raise tension and make it much more difficult to handle. So, improving your assertiveness will enable you to boost your self-esteem. Often it will help to improve self-belief by behaving as though you believe in yourself!

- Enhance your physical fitness

Whenever we are active and balanced, it is much better to feel great about ourselves. People with poor self-esteem, nevertheless, often ignore themselves as they don't believe they deserve to be taken care of.

Try to do some workouts, have a decent meal, and get adequate sleep. It's equally a great idea to create time to rest and do other things you like to do, instead of what someone else has forced you to do. You might find simple improvements like this could make a big difference to your current situation.

- Take on challenges

Individuals with low self-esteem usually avoid complicated and intimidating circumstances. In reality, taking on a challenge could be one method of raising your self-esteem. This does not imply that you have to do it yourself. Part of the challenge may be to request aid anytime you need it, though be ready to attempt things you aware would be challenging to accomplish.

By thriving, you prove yourself that you are capable of achieving a lot. This challenges your negative feelings and will raise your self-esteem as a result.

The Significance of Baby Steps

It is quite doubtful that suddenly you'll go from bad to positive self-esteem. Instead, over some time, you would definitely find that you are making incremental changes. The trick is to consider the long term, instead of day-to-day, and concentrate on the long view, not the specifics of how you felt at a specific period yesterday.

If you feel positive or do something great, enjoy it, but if you sometimes fall back into negative thought habits, don't tear yourself up. Only pick yourself up again and strive to be more optimistic in your thought. This will gradually become a habit, and you will realize that your self-esteem has steadily improved.

Chapter 13: INSTANT MOTIVATION

The Myth of Motivation

If you watch every professional sports event, you will find outstanding athletes flop irrespective of the months of preparation. It doesn't matter how fantastic they were a week ago or even yesterday. They may have a lot of expertise, highly great skills, and the right resources, but does this ensure an outstanding performance? All the proof indicates that it doesn't, and in any other field, we also see several indications of this.

So if it's not expertise and experience, what is the actual determinant in the desire to succeed? What helps you to thrive and remain calm in the center of the storm amidst obstacles? What motivates you to do what's right?

There is no question that it is important to be in a good state of mind and feel motivated, positive, and committed to doing our best. Yet, there is one underlying misconception that this chapter seeks to fix when it comes to succeeding at work. It refers to the critical role that motivation plays in our thought and what determines our professional life's success.

I recall watching Andy Murray perform in 2012 at Wimbledon. He was a professional player on the court, slipping down on his performance. He had the expertise and abilities to steal the show, although it actually came down to when it was played. You could see him becoming increasingly more frustrated, and his game declined as his frustration grew. He came back with a new mentality the next year, and he won Wimbledon.

Outside the world of sport, what is the actual determinant you can get a range of responses, including self-confidence, previous experience, great relationships, excellent working environment, effective leadership, the right talents? The alternatives are many and varied.

Likewise, whenever you ask people what sabotages or de-motivates them at work, you'll hear various explanations, such as pressure, bad management, insufficient time, strict schedules, or too much tension, to mention a few. To many individuals, it appears as if their ups and downs have many reasons. However, the underlying issue is tied to their motivation and sense of focus on their professional goal. You'll learn a few strategies to shift your motivation instantly from rookie to expert.

The Role of Motivation in the Quest for Success

- It raises the energy levels

Whenever you are inspired, your whole body is filled with adrenaline to enable you to achieve the targets you have set for yourself, resulting in increased energy levels. For instance, you seldom become tired once you're enthusiastic about a task you're working on. And you can enjoy all night long without any issues when you're out drinking. However, if you were taking a yoga class that you hated, on the contrary, you'd be struggling to get through an hour. We immediately watch our energy levels increasing as we have control over our tasks and priorities, as we are more concentrated and enthusiastic about the outcome. This shows that motivation for work will increase our levels of energy and help us to perform better.

- It will make you happy

Motivation creates a desire to do something, such as attending a training session or securing a new contract, and you feel satisfied with your results whenever you progress. So, if you keep inspiring yourself and setting and reaching new goals, you will typically feel better than you have done before.

And while achievement is the source of motivation, satisfaction is the fundamental desire that drives motivation. So, set yourself tiny goals and learn to be happy with incremental progress to ensure that your satisfaction and motivational levels increase. I shall talk more about this later

- It's contagious

It's bound to rub off on their peers if one team member is inspired, allowing more workers to be dedicated and guided. Indeed, one Sandglaz Blog research reveals that 'whenever a group member feels and expresses positive emotions, others are more inclined to react favorably to that team member's social impact attempts.' This is important to your personal life as well. Reflect on the time you spent with a positive person; did they rub off their positive energy on you and cause you to feel more productive? If so, remember how your positive energy will affect those around you and, as a result, make them feel more inspired.

- It improves your results

According to Dr. Anders Ericsson's study, and as Jim Taylor, Ph.D., reports in Psychology Today, motivation is the most important success indicator, and success is accomplished through high performance. You can inherently be a great worker by knowing what inspires you to do better, move up the life ladder quicker, or achieve your professional goals. Researchers at Cornell University, Kaitlin Woolley and Ayelet Fishbach, observed in recent research published in the Journal of Personality and Social Psychology that 'offering individuals an instant reward for completing a task, instead of holding until the end of the task to reward them, increased their participation and satisfaction in the task.'

- It increases your devotion

Individuals get more devoted to the mission and put all their energy into it if they are inspired to do anything. When you're instinctively inspired to do a great job, it sounds simple, but whenever you're feeling demoralized, you need to remember the value of devotion to your overall performance. Let's assume you're looking for a promotion in your job. If you are driven and dedicated to doing the best you can, you would have a great chance of grabbing the promotion and progressing in your career.

- It allows you to handle your time more effectively.

To deal with the difficulties that the world throws at us and do so effectively, motivation is necessary. For instance, highly motivated individuals are structured, and they assign set times to various tasks in their plans, giving themselves a predetermined time to complete each one. Many that are less inspired, on the contrary, do not adhere to a particular schedule and end up procrastinating in the process. Anything easy, like getting up for work and waking up early, is a perfect example. You'll be better inspired to get out of bed and work on time if you enjoy what you do. However, if you appear dissatisfied, you might end up hitting the 'Snooze' key a few times and spending excessive time in the process.

- It lets you grow as a person.

Motivation promotes the growth of oneself. Indeed, you will feel more motivated to drive yourself harder and accomplish greater things when you set your personal goals and you achieve them.

Take Rihanna, for example, who began singing when she was 17 years old. She has since starred in blockbuster films, including Ocean 8 and Valerian and the City of a Thousand Worlds, and has launched a lingerie company and her makeup brand. She's gained tremendous success by continuing to set herself new goals and has developed herself as an entertainer and entrepreneur.

- It builds faith in yourself.

People who lack trust usually are afraid of getting out of their comfort zone and doing something new. However, you would have a small chance of success if you do not take risks. This doesn't necessarily mean that to try anything different. You need to drop your whole routine. Instead, before you know what you love and what keeps you going, you can juggle a few different duties on the go. If you're thinking of starting up your own company, for example, start while you're still working. If you can see that it's successful, then it's a solid sign to quit your day job and concentrate exclusively on your business. However, you'll have the safety net of your career to fall back on if it's not going as expected.

Success is unachievable without inspiration. And while success is the vision, it's important to note that happiness is what is most important in the equation because there would be no sense of meaning for your accomplishment without happiness.

Strategies Used In Developing Instant Motivation

- Don't think of it as an impossible task

For me, there is solely one way of motivating myself to accomplish a task: I don't think of it as an impossible task. I believe it is part of turning myself into the kind of person I wish to be. I try not to worry too much about how hard or stressful or impossible it could be once I have decided to embark on a course of action or a task; I think about how amazing it would feel to be something or how pleased I could be to have achieved that. Make the impossible look easy.

As Marie Stein put it. Think about it: if the task you're facing is not seen as drudgery but instead as a piece of the puzzle that helps you towards your professional path, then it would be easier to get the motivation needed to do it.

- Set tiny, bite-sized goals

There's an explanation why donut holes are so endearing. They're quick to consume. You've consumed a couple of them before you know it. This is the manner priorities set, too. You ought to have a very high, ambitious goal. However, make sure you split the goal down into consumable, bite-sized targets. In this manner, as you achieve the smaller tasks, you will feel like you are making progress on your quest, and you will also feel a sense of achievement. A sense of success and accomplishment is a lovely mix of effective motivation.

You've, without a doubt, came across this advice before, but did you apply it to motivation? It is difficult to complete a massive job task you have no idea of where to begin. When you have no clue where you're starting, how can you complete the task? But instead of concentrating on a huge, frightening target, take one thing at a time and split the big target into ideas that you can absorb one at a time."

- Read Daily

Be ready to take out some time to read in your day. (I suggest the early mornings before anyone is up.) Read for a minimum of one hour per day. If that appears to be too much, begin with 30 minutes [per day] and try this for one month (habit). Establish a conviction that the fastest way to excel is to learn. This will render reading a breeze and incredibly fun/rewarding (if you're motivated by success). The world's most prominent individuals owe their achievement to reading some books (Warren Buffet, Bill Gates, Elon Musk).

Though setting aside a reading period can appear counterintuitive when what you are searching for is the motivation for a set task, it is sometimes important to consider something largely disparate to handle the task at hand. One thing that's sure to have a long-lasting effect on your thinking processes is forming a daily reading habit, eventually motivating you in all aspects of life.

- Avoid thinking about things that do not matter.

It costs you a lot of mental resources to do stuff that doesn't mean anything. Check your extensive to-do list, identify tasks you think you don't care for or have little to no significance, and get rid of as much of these tasks as you can. If you are working on intrinsically important tasks or are part of a broader goal, you will be more regularly inspired.

Look through your list critically and objectively, and cut off everything you need to do that is both genuinely demotivating and redundant. It's not usually best to complete what you began if, down the line, you are not able to recall the purpose you started it in the first instance.

- Set a Time to quit

Business people prefer to stray from the traditional working days of 8 to 5, and it is more than convenient to provide a 24-hour workday via global accessibility using mails and Skype. However, understanding when enough is crucial. Define for yourself a practical quitting time, and adhere to it most times of the week. Right after 8 PM, stop replying to emails, or take Saturdays and Sundays off. Once you give yourself some downtime, you'll seem more relaxed and more motivated.

Put up your hand if you're motivated 24/7! It's impractical to feel motivated every time, to wish to plow through assignments all the time. You have to offer yourself a break, and if that implies giving yourself a given fixed time to disconnect or look away from your work's needs, then do it. This will likely make you function better and more intelligently in the hours that you allocate for work.

- Simply do it

From my personal experience, the most powerful strategy for me to be motivated to begin doing something is just doing it (it appears ordinary, but it works). You feel you have to do something immediately, jump straight at it, and do it instantly (surely, provided the conditions are feasible). You ought not to think about any other thing, to erase all other emotions, to keep your mind clean, to behave like a machine. Yeah, it seems strange, but it works! Otherwise, you can discuss if you can do it now or whether there have been so many difficulties doing it, or whether there are more pleasant and interesting other things to do over this tedious job.

So here's a few valuable pieces of advice: Rather than sitting around, hoping to feel inspired, what if you simply went on and start doing the job you know you have to do? Jump straight into the task and believe that the concentration you will be what you require.

- Start celebrating wins

Start to remember all the positive things you are doing. Don't underestimate the tiny stuff. How frequently, I mean, are you scolding yourself for doing something tiny that wasn't great? How much do you feel the positive things like being on time or signing a new deal is actually how it supposed to be? They require celebrating. In your career, you need more wins. This will inspire you, empower you, and make you see how brilliant you are.

You forget how important all the small wins are if you're continually looking for a long-term reward. And keeping focused and on top of the situation could be difficult if there's no payoff in view. Treat yourself with small things and do not overlook how satisfying it can feel to celebrate small achievements.

Chapter 14: QUICK PROBLEM-SOLVING

Every day everyone has to make decisions, and we all face a myriad of challenges that need solving. Whether the problem is large or small, we all set targets for ourselves, face obstacles and work to solve them.

Whenever you can solve problems by providing easy solutions, your ability as a professional immediately increases. It's essential to mention that being a problem solver isn't simply a skill; it's a whole mindset, one that enables individuals to bring out the best in themselves, so be very focused on your journey.

Problem-solving is simple whenever you know how to do it efficiently. Your aim as a professional should be to transform problem-solving into practice so that you feel more motivated when potential problems arise.

You will feel accomplished by the problems you solve. You deal with problems that may otherwise seem massive, daunting, or overly complex to others. Your manner of viewing things, your mode of thinking, is special, and it is founded upon your own experiences, mistakes, and achievement. That's what you need. You follow a concise shortcut to problem-solving. You progress by moving away from barriers hindering your development, and you steer yourself in the right direction for success.

To be an efficient problem-solver, you have to be strategic and rational at the same time. Whenever you solve problems, you enable yourself to make more successful decisions that will benefit your personal or professional development. And as you improve your problem-solving abilities, you equally increase your confidence and value as a professional.

Everyone will gain from having strong problem-solving skills as we all face problems regularly. Most of these challenges are more serious or complicated than others. It would be great to solve all problems easily and promptly without struggle. Sadly, there is no one approach where all problems can be solved. As you browse through this chapter on problem-solving, you will find that the topic is complex.

However well trained we are towards problem-solving, there is still an aspect of the unknown. While preparation and organizing will hopefully make the problem-solving approach more probable to be effective, good judgment and an amount of good fortune will ultimately decide whether problem-solving was a success.

Professionals, Interpersonal relationships, and companies fail because of inadequate problem-solving skills. This is primarily due to either concern not being understood or being identified but not being appropriately addressed.

Sports experts widely value problem-solving skills, war soldiers, and employers as many businesses rely on their workers to identify and solve problems.

A ton of the activity in problem-solving requires knowing the root causes of the problem, not the signs. Attempting to handle a customer complaint should be seen as a problem that has to be addressed, and it's almost definitely a great idea to do so. The person handling the dissatisfaction should be wondering what has prompted the customer to query in the first place. If the source of the dissatisfaction can be resolved, then the problem is solved.

Skills Needed for Effective Problem-Solving

To be successful at problem-solving, you are going to need several other primary skills, which include:

- **Creativity**

Problems are typically solved either instinctively or manually. Instinct is used whenever no new insight is required - you understand enough to make a fast decision, fix the problems, or apply common sense or wisdom to address the problem. You have not faced highly complicated problems or problems before will definitely take a more organized and rational approach to manage them. For these, you will have to apply imaginative thinking.

- **Researching Abilities**

Identifying and solving problems also needs you to do some analysis: this could be a quick Google keyword search or more comprehensive research on the concept.

- **Team Working**

Most problems, especially office and military problems, are better described and addressed with other individuals' support. Team working can appear like a 'job thing,' but it is simply as critical at home and school and in the workplace.

- **Emotional Intelligence**

It is important to remember the effect that a problem and its remedy have on you and other individuals. Emotional intelligence, the capacity to recognize yourself and other people's feelings, can help direct you to an acceptable solution.

- **Risk Management**

Fixing a problem requires a fair level of risk - this risk must be assessed appropriately against not fixing the problem.

- **Decision Making**

Problem-solving and decision making are strongly linked concepts, and making a decision is an essential aspect of the problem-solving process as you will always be presented with multiple choices and options

Stages Involved in Problem-Solving

Generally, successful problem solving requires going through a series of steps or phases, such as those listed below.

- **Problem Identification**

This stage entails: recognizing and accepting that a problem exists, establishing the existence of the problem, defining the problem.

The first step of problem-solving can sound simple, but further thought and research are often needed. Identifying a problem can, in itself, be a challenging job. Is there a problem at all? What is the essence of the problem? Are there multiple problems? How is it possible to better define the problem? You will not only comprehend it more explicitly yourself but will be able to explain its complexity to others by taking quality time describing the problem, which moves us to the second step.

- **Structuring the Problem**

This stage includes a time of observation, thorough inspection, fact-searching, and creating a realistic image of the issue.

Following on from problem recognition, designing the problem is all about obtaining more problem knowledge and growing comprehension. This step is all about discovering and evaluating evidence, providing a more accurate image of both the objective(s) and the obstacle (s). For very clear problems, this stage may not be appropriate, but it is important for problems of a more complicated nature.

- **Searching for Possible Ideas**

You will create some potential courses of action during this process, but at this point, with little attempt to analyze them.

It is now time to begin thinking about potential remedies to the defined problem from the knowledge collected in the first two phases of the problem-solving process. This stage is sometimes conducted as a brain-storming exercise in a group situation like the military case, allowing each person in the group to share their views on potential solutions. Different persons will have different experiences in various organizations, and it is also valuable to seek each individual's opinions.

- **Making Decision**

This process entails careful consideration of the various potential courses of action and then selecting the appropriate execution solution.

This is maybe the most difficult aspect of the method of problem-solving. Following the preceding step, it is now time to reflect on and critically examine each possible solution. Due to other issues, such as time limits or budgets, certain solutions might not be feasible. At this stage, it is equally important to consider what could happen if nothing was done to address the problem. Sometimes, it takes some very innovative thinking and great ideas to try to solve a problem that could result in many more problems.

Lastly, it is imperative to decide which course of action to take as decision-making is a critical ability in itself.

- **Implementation**

This stage includes accepting the desired course of action and implementing it. Implementation implies acting on the solution selected. Many more problems may surface during implementation, particularly if identifying or structuring the initial problem was not conducted carefully.

- **Monitoring/Seeking Feedback**

The final stage is about evaluating the results of problem-solving over a long period, which includes eliciting feedback as to the progress of the results of the selected solution.

The last stage of problem-solving is concerned with verifying that the process is effective. This can be done by monitoring and acquiring feedback from individuals affected by any developments that happened. It is a great practice to maintain a record of results and any issues that arise.

Strategies Used In Problem-Solving

There are a variety of different ways in which individuals solve a problem. A few of these strategies may be applied independently, but individuals may also employ some methods to find out and solve a problem.

- **Algorithms**

An algorithm is a step-by-step process that produces the perfect solution at all times. A mathematical model is a great example of an algorithm for problem-solving. While an algorithm ensures a correct answer, it is not usually the best problem-solving strategy.

For certain cases, this approach is not realistic because it can be too time-consuming. For starters, if you were attempting to use an algorithm to work out all the potential number arrangements for a lock, this would consume a very large amount of time.

- **Heuristics**

A heuristic is a strategy of cognitive rule-of-thumb that in some circumstances can or may not apply. Heuristics do not usually guarantee the right solution, unlike algorithms.

Nevertheless, applying this problem-solving technique makes it possible for individuals to solve difficult problems and minimize the total number of potential solutions to a more achievable range.

- **Trial and Error**

A problem-solving trial-and-error strategy requires pursuing various approaches and leaving out those that do not fit. When you have a tiny number of potential options, this strategy can be a great choice.

If there are several distinct alternatives, you are better off filtering down the potential solutions using another problem-solving strategy before trying trial-and-error.

- **Insight**

The solution to a problem will emerge as a spontaneous insight into certain circumstances. This may happen when you know that something you have previously worked with is similar to the problem. Nevertheless, outside of consciousness, the essential cognitive processes that result in insight happen.

Common Obstacles in Problem-Solving

Problem-solving is definitely, not a seamless operation. Various obstacles can conflict with our capacity to rapidly and effectively solve a problem. A range of such mental barriers has been identified by experts that include functional fixedness, insignificant knowledge, and assumptions.

Assumptions

Individuals sometimes make assumptions whenever they are faced with a problem about the limitations and barriers that prohibit those solutions.

Functional Fixedness

This concept refers to the propensity to see problems only in their normal form. Functional fixedness stops an individual from completely seeing any of the multiple choices available to reach a solution.

Insignificant or Deceptive knowledge

It is crucial to differentiate between knowledge that is significant to the problem and insignificant information that can result in incorrect solutions while you are attempting to solve a problem. When a problem is really complicated, it's easier to concentrate on inaccurate or insignificant results.

Mental set

A mental set tends to apply only strategies that have succeeded in the past instead of searching for alternative ideas.

A mental set may also serve as a heuristic, making it a valuable resource for problem-solving. Mental set, nevertheless, can equally contribute to rigidity, making it harder to find successful solutions.

Chapter 15: THINKING CLEARER, SMARTER & FASTER

It is reported that 75 percent of individuals are afraid of public speaking. But digging further, it could also be that individuals are unable to think quickly in those circumstances. Looking further than that, there are probably all categories of other social events in which you desire you could think quickly. From developing witty remarks to completing a task more quickly, thinking quickly has different advantages and needs the training to accomplish it.

The significance of Fast Thinking

We have to understand why it's essential before we master how crucial it is. If there is no purpose of practicing, then, after a while, we will eventually stop. Having the ability to think fast offers a wide range of advantages.:

- People are going to think you're smarter.
- They are extremely happy, more innovative, full of energy, and self-confident whenever people are asked to think fast.
- Fast thinking also relates to organizing, problem-solving, setting objectives, and being able to concentrate.
- Also, quicker thinking will keep your brain intellectually stimulated.

- You're going to experience faster response time as well.

The list is comprehensive. However, the concept is that the stronger your brain is, the more it can be used in many fields of life.

How Fast Do You Think?

How does one improve thinking speed is the next question? The response is through a number of methods that I have mentioned below:

- Make small decisions faster

Over the day, we're confronted with several decisions. However, some of them are not as essential as others. Food is vital, although it is irrelevant to decide between a sandwich, burger, or haggis. Being able to determine what to eat easily will allow you to think quicker.

After all, the implications are minimal, even if your choice wasn't the right one. This practice works as this is simply the act of thinking quickly.

But one thing I'm trying to emphasize with this advice is the keyword, minor decisions. In more critical life-changing choices that will have greater consequences, never apply this strategy.

- Practice Speed

There's much stuff that we try every time, which we have become very good at, playing music, practicing songs, reading, or doing particular stretches. Whatever the situation, I motivate you to add another aspect of the challenge to those abilities through speeding up. Similar to the technique above, this often requires that you think quickly to execute a mission.

A timer would help you practice speed—time to complete a business assignment or run a lap on your own. To accomplish a task, you may assign yourself an allocated time.

This second approach is remarkably productive since the most critical aspects of that task would be automatically prioritized by most individuals. It's called the Law of Parkinsons.

- Stop Multitasking

We just can't, as much as we'd like to believe we can complete numerous tasks altogether. Our mind, as strong as it is, is unable to concentrate on two activities at once. But why are people allowed to rub their tummies and pat their heads?

Yeah, that's because our mind flips between tasks quickly. In those cases, the minds of individuals switch more easily between those tasks. However, outside of those cases, the study discovered that multitasking decreases the period of concentration, our capacity to learn, and our cognitive efficiency. Consequently, prioritizing a single task and giving it our full attention before completion is smarter for us.

- Get Enough Sleep

Sufficient sleep is not solely required for body function but also cognitive ability. One research discovered that not sleeping properly would affect the speed and precision of our thought. It makes sense, by that rationale, that sleep would help keep our brains healthy and more efficient.

- Meditate

Another approach for us to relax our minds is daily meditation. All sorts of research have been done demonstrating how meditation enables us to build new brain cells and neural circuits. That's because meditation enhances contact between cells in the first place.

- Do physical exercise

To a certain extent, all exercise is good for us and our brains. That being said, physical activities have clearly been shown to increase our brain's processing capability. Activities such as jogging, cycling, riding, and swimming are physical exercises.

Strategies Used In Clear Thinking

- Check your attitude

How our attention suits our impulses is unbelievable. To explain this, check how simple it is to think of many ways and new ideas to accomplish a target whenever you want it. Contrarily, note how you concentrate on all the reasons why it is not a great idea to step forward if you do not want to accomplish a goal. Try to be frank about your motivation to accomplish a specific purpose to achieve a simple focus. Do you want it? At the very beginning, this can save you a great deal of time or your efforts.

- Have a definite purpose

We must be precise to accomplish our objectives. The reasoning for this is that thinking about a moving goal is difficult. If we continue to change our target, we ask our brain to change its emphasis and lose our course constantly. Sit down for five minutes to retain your concentration and write down what you intend to accomplish as simply as you can.

- Use your enthusiasm to manage your feelings

There is a clear explanation why this is so: Enthusiasm conquers challenges as it focuses on the joy of reaching the ultimate result as you aim for your objective. Your feelings, nevertheless, may be overcome by issues when they feel the pain of a possible loss of the goal to the Ego.

Think forward clearly to accomplish what you desire to maintain your concentration: use your enthusiasm to control your feelings.

- use your negative thinking to produce a positive outcome

Our negative thinking is one of the most important abilities we have. Far from negative thinking that contributes to resentment, negative thinking is the catalyst that can enable our creativity to do just what we desire.

You can encourage your imagination to channel your negative thoughts into constructive action by using the expression 'Why not = How to'?

Anna, a founder of a large company in the UK, stated how, by using this strategy, she was able to advance her career internationally.

- Using Cool Reasoning in Hot Situations

Ensures that you steer all discussions objectively and intentionally to advance the objective you desire to achieve.

Mastering these five basic strategies will turn your psychology into what you want to achieve.

Chapter 16: ACHIEVING FRUITFUL EFFECTIVENESS

Do you see yourself at work as being effective? While many of us would like to believe that we are 100 percent effective, the fact is that we all have strengths and weaknesses that impair our ability to be effective. Most of us could profit from fine-tuning at least a few of our abilities in order to boost our effectiveness. Maybe you've often flourished at time management, for example. However, how much time do you devote to learning new skills and keeping up with business trends and work demands?

Or, perhaps you're good at handling the substantial demands that you face every day. Though when things get very intense, your communication skills tend to suffer as your stress levels increase. Now and across our careers, being fruitfully effective at work will pay off. Successful employees receive exciting projects, acquire large customers, and their colleagues and managers are well regarded. But how can you become more effective and ensure that such fantastic opportunities are not missed? And what should you concentrate on?

This is what we're going to talk about in this chapter. To become more effective, we will look at the abilities you can improve, and we will examine strategies and tools you may use to maximize your effectiveness.

Step 1: Set Your Priorities

Would you have a reasonable answer if someone asked you what your work was really about? Knowing your intent at work is one of the most important steps in being effective. After all, how can you set acceptable goals if you don't understand what your work is meant to accomplish? (You'll be trapped under a huge amount of tasks forever if you don't set goals, unable to make the distinction between what's relevant and what isn't.)

Perform a career review to assess your job's true intent and decide what you have to accomplish in your current position. This will help you discover your most crucial priorities so that you may effectively begin prioritizing activities.

Step 2: Keep a Good Mindset

There's a "positive mindset" for all effective professionals. But what exactly does this imply? Individuals with a positive mindset take the initiative when they do. They support a partner in need enthusiastically. They take up the shift when someone is off sick and ensure their job is completed to the best expectations. "Good enough" is never quite good enough for them!

More than just winning your respect, a positive attitude at work would do more: setting standards for your job and your actions implies you take responsibility for yourself. In certain institutions, this valuable quality is difficult to come by. Although showing sensible decision and honesty could, in the long-term, unlocks many doors for you.

As a result, concentrate on keeping a positive mindset at work and making choices that "ring true" instinctively. You'll sleep better at night at the very least!

Step 3: Develop Crucial Skills

The odds are that on your time, you have a lot of growing demands. Learning to handle your time more effectively is one of the most important ways to improve your work effectiveness. Mastering how to handle stress, developing communication skills, and taking action on career development are other main areas. Both of these can have a massive impact on your job effectiveness.

Let's take a closer look at each skill.

Time Management

Learning to control your time is perhaps the most important thing you can do to increase your work effectiveness. Your days will seem like a chaotic sprint without this expertise, with every project, text, and phone call vying for your attention.

Begin by taking a good look at your daily routine. Do you realize how you spend all your time each day? If not, you may be shocked by the answer! To determine how much time you spend on your different activities, such as meetings, workouts, training sessions, checking emails, making phone calls, and using event logs. Looking at this critically can be an eye-opening process, particularly if you realize that you spend a lot of time on activities that don't help you reach your goals.

When you realize how much time you commit to various activities, you have to prioritize them. You would be able to concentrate on the tasks that offer the most benefit if you recognize which tasks are critical and which could be delayed or delegated—using a professional resource like a To-Do List or (better still) an Action Plan to keep records of it all to ensure that you do not neglect important tasks and duties.

Being effective at work entails making the most of your time. Plan your work of greatest importance for the times of day when you are the most efficient. This raises the chances that while working, you can resist disturbances and reach a state of balance.

Goal Setting

Another essential part of working effectively is goal setting. You ought to have a good understanding of what your position is all about once you've done a Job Review. Apply this information to set short and long-term objectives. The benefit of doing so is that your ambitions serve as a road map. After all, if you don't know where you're heading, you'll never get there!

Working fruitfully and effectively requires good organization as well. You can spend a massive amount of time just searching for missing things if you're disorganized. So, master how to file correctly and how to make a plan that works for you.

Communication

Reflect on just how much we communicate every day. We make telephone calls, attend meetings, focus group discussions, brainstorming, write letters, give presentations, speak to clients, etc. We may appear to spend the whole day conversing with those around us. This is why, particularly when your aim is to function more effectively, strong communication skills are important. Begin by honing your active listening abilities. This suggests that you are putting in a deliberate effort to hear and comprehend what others are saying to you genuinely.

Don't get bothered by what's happening around you, and don't formulate your following words while the other individual is speaking. Instead, pay attention to what they're doing. You would be shocked how much miscommunication can be prevented just by consciously listening. Next, check your writing skills. How well do you express yourself in writing? Starting with your inbox. Every day, the majority of us send thousands of emails. But there are several approaches we can use to make sure that we write productive emails that are read!

When preparing an email, for example, stick to one key subject. It would be challenging for your partner to prioritize and sort the data by putting multiple significant topics in one message. If you must bring up numerous points, label them consecutively or break them into different messages with related subject keywords. We do a lot more writing, of course, than just text. We communicate through instant messaging, write reports, and build presentations. You'll be more efficient in your job if you learn to connect more effectively through all of these channels, and your boss and coworkers will certainly appreciate your efforts, as they'll be the primary beneficiaries!

Stress

A small amount of pressure may be helpful. When stress exceeds your ability to deal with it efficiently, however, your productivity suffers, as does your mood. You may lose the capacity to make sound, reasonable decisions, and, both in the short and long term, constant stress may cause health problems. Whatever you do, you'll almost definitely face stress at some stage during your career, maybe even daily. This is why learning how to cope with stress is vital to be more effective at work.

Make an effort to get a decent night's rest every day, and stop bringing work home with you. Whenever you get home at night, it is also important to relax. Keep a stress log for a week or more if you're not certain what causes the stress. It allows you to recognize the things that trigger your stress and recognize the extent to which you feel it. You can then evaluate these stimuli when you feel relaxed and develop successful methods for handling them.

Learning/Professional Development

No matter what your profession is, you must continue to learn and improve your skills. To define the areas you need to work on, conduct a Personal SWOT Analysis. You must concentrate on soft skills in addition to the technical skills required for your work. Leadership skills, problem-solving strategies, emotional intelligence skills, and imaginative thinking are among them. Any attempt you make to develop these abilities will pay off in the workplace.

Chapter 17: GREATER EFFICIENCY

At the end of the workday, how many of you have glanced up at the clock and thought like you really didn't get enough done? Are you working from home or on your journey and still unable to achieve your objectives? Why is it that you have not yet figured out how to boost job efficiency? Designing a more organized and efficient method of handling your work-related tasks not only increases your efficiency, but it equally allows you more free time to do whatever you want about it, whether it's improving yourself or relaxing.

To better evaluate and incorporate efficiency improvements into current business processes, business professionals must first know the idea of workplace efficiency. Efficiency is characterized as the process that yields the best output using the smallest amount of resources. Working efficiently leads to higher volume output from the same resource input quantity.

Efficiency in the working environment typically describes an individual employee's activities and labor in a single workday. The concept of workplace efficiency includes activities and work done by a team or department. In order to be considered efficient, an individual must work tirelessly and deliberately to complete their tasks.

Efficient individuals usually:

- Complete assignments based on priority
- Break up projects into assignments and assignments into subtasks
- Take short, regular breaks
- Distract themself as least as possible.
- Purposefully communicate
- Delegate Mindfully

Expanding your work efficiency involves the same time and effort as every other self-improvement initiative. Rather than detracting from it, you are ultimately developing new habits that will lead to your productivity. To get you started, here are some strategies:

Strategies Used In Boosting Career Efficiency

- Change Your Time Management Strategy

You may have to develop your time management skills if you find yourself immersed in work, moving from task to task without a simple plan, or coping with work performance. To feel less stressed and more coordinated, acquaint yourself with chunking practices, which group tasks together based on the result. If you're applying chunking to plan your day, you could put tasks like responding to emails and returning phone calls at the beginning of the day, when you're fresher, and errands that don't take much thought, like picking up pet food, at the end.

When you increase your efficiency by time management skills, you decrease anxiety and achieve more, creating a cycle that helps you to accomplish even more.

- Ditch Digital Devices

We spend much of our day looking at some kind of computer. Although heavy computer usage may be part of your work, digital devices can be a big diversion, and social media sites can also harm your wellbeing. By walking away from your mobile or device, increase your work efficiency. At a meeting, consider taking written notes to see if your ideas flow more freely. There's nothing particularly wrong with digital devices, but presenting yourself with a slight break from your usual processes will push your mind to function in new, productive ways. You might also find that when you write something down by hand rather than typing it on a screen, your memory improves.

Detach yourself from the Internet or turn off your social media if you're being interrupted by social networks or other websites and have to use your computer to get work done. When you can't quickly turn to Facebook or another intrusive website, you can concentrate on the task at hand and improve productivity dramatically.

When you can't easily turn to Facebook or other distracting websites, you can concentrate on the task at hand and improve productivity dramatically. Another way to boost efficiency at work is to keep your phone out of reach and on silent when working on a project – imagine how much more you could get done without browsing through mobile applications or being tempted to share vacation plans with your friends family.

- Teach Yourself to Say "No"

We often take on things we shouldn't have to, whether it's because we feel pressure from ourselves or people around us. We're so concentrated on demonstrating the multitasking skills that we assume roles that we could simply as easily delegate to others. We equate the word "No" with missed chances or failure, but that's not at all the case. When your plate is already full, or you just lack confidence in a job, learn how to say no. Do so if you can delegate smaller duties to those around you. Relieving yourself from your schedule helps you concentrate more closely on things that actually matter to you and boost job performance.

- Take a break from time to time

Are you having trouble coming up with a good idea? Feeling like you've got so much homework, you don't know where to start? Worrying that you have so much to do can be a cognitive barrier in and of itself. You'll have spent a day excruciating about what to do first or how to get it accomplished before you know it. That is an easy way to do nothing.

Pause for a moment. Do something entirely unconnected to the task at hand. Go on a stroll. Do a little meditation. Play some songs. Energy flows where the emphasis goes, and if your concentration is trapped on a task that you can't even make any progress on, your energy is disrupted, and work performance ceases. Shifting your concentration will improve your situation, so you feel fresh and energized to approach your task with a fresh mind when you return to work. Over your workday, plan in frequent breaks to allow yourself time to rest and reorganize, and you will find that work efficiency improves naturally.

- Establishing a routine that you enjoy

Individuals who regularly achieve their objectives by increasing work efficiency do so by cultivating long-term behaviors. Build a routine that helps you to be as efficient as possible at work. Everybody's routine looks unique, so find the one that makes you feel the greatest. Every morning, you can end up at the gym for an hour or take a long walk at lunch to relieve some tension. Understanding the link between mind and body can allow you to see that not only does a conscious priming exercise help you boost effectiveness, but it can also enable you to unlock an exceptional life. Your work performance can skyrocket if you develop a routine that makes you feel comfortable, safe, and clear-headed.

- Let Go of Perfection

Perfection is a misconception that creates tension and can lead to restrictions discouraging you from achieving your full potential. Seek Knowledge and understanding that nothing is ever going to be accomplished perfectly. It also allows you to see failures as opportunities for growth; once you stop fearing failure, you'll be less likely to procrastinate, as we often put stuff off to prevent trying and failing.

Listen to and change your self-talk and reduce perfectionism. Treat yourself with dignity and allow yourself some leeway if you don't always meet your self-imposed high expectations. When you let go of perfectionism and just concentrate on growth, your productivity and overall well-being will increase.

- Improve the environment

It's not all about the environment when it comes to learning how to maximize productivity at work. Do you find yourself sandwiched between two chatty coworkers? Will you have to leave your office daily to pick up printouts or make copies? Is your desk a jumbled mess that makes you feel nervous as soon as you walk in the door? Next, look at how your room is fun and inspiring. Do you have some music playing that inspires you? Is there any artwork on the walls that makes you happy? Improving job productivity necessitates a conducive work setting. Consider consulting with an interior designer or practical workplace consultant for guidance if you're unsure how to make your office more conducive to your job.

CONCLUSION

Are you the kind of person in your life who needs to achieve huge success? Will you have the emotional fortitude to pull it off? Achieving success can be challenging no matter your aspirations, and over time, the daily routine can take its toll on your physical, mental, and emotional energy. Failure, fatigue, discouragement, exhaustion, self-limiting convictions, tension, and so much more await achievers and high performers from all walks of life on their journey to success.

However, how do some individuals, year after year, consistently work for their personal goals while others give up on them? How do those individuals, when too much is stacked against them, remain powerful and persevere? A key to performance is mental toughness. the key to outstanding achievement is not talent, but a rare mixture of zeal and perseverance known as 'grit.'" In other words, when it comes to reaching goals, mental toughness is key.

Mentally tough individuals can overcome these challenges and find a path to success, while those with low mental toughness often give up on their dreams. Build a positive mentality. The first thing you have to do is work on creating a solid, optimistic attitude in daily life if you're going to improve your mental strength and handle stress.

Carrying negative feelings around with you is like going on a mountain hike with a backpack full of rocks. The hike is hard enough on its own, but a prescription for failure is to have extra junk weighing you down. Building mental resilience isn't only about adding new strength and reserving the current strength for the right tasks. Instead of struggling to get big enough to bear the extra weight, wouldn't it be better to empty the backpack's rocks? Let go of self-limiting convictions. When you're always beating yourself up, it's very hard to be mentally tough. Any values that hold you back in any way are self-limiting beliefs.

Negative self-talk runs wild when we encourage these self-limiting views to flood our minds, and we crowd out our ability to think positively. When you find a self-limiting conviction emerging in your mind, quickly silence it by reminding yourself that it isn't real, followed by some optimistic affirmations.

Self-limiting values and an all-or-nothing mentality will lead to a bad case of dwelling on the negative, which is bad mental health news. You have to ditch the dwelling if you want to develop some mental toughness and keep your mind strong. When we focus on our misfortunes, we waste many resources that could be better spent on achieving our objectives. We're more likely to leave entirely when this happens.

Allow yourself to feel disappointed and angry the next time anything bad happens, but focus on that the amount of time you concentrate on the situation. Find a way to communicate with your goal. Having a good "why" for both of your short and long-term goals is one of the most crucial aspects of improving mental toughness and maintaining a strong and concentrated mind. Suppose you set out to accomplish a big target for which you don't have a "why," you'll become distracted, frustrated, or disengaged as soon as you meet the first setback.

Find Power in Peace. The final element of gaining mental toughness is to accept the fact that you're not alone in this. You must know that you do not have to go it alone to develop unrivaled mental toughness. A team backs up even the toughest Navy Seals. Learn to pick yourself up after losses. It is not easy to build a positive mentality and grow mental toughness! Obstacles, failures, and disappointment are unavoidable for anyone who has ever achieved massive success, and you are no exception.

You will face many ups and downs while you focus on your goals, but this doesn't mean you don't have mental resilience, willpower, or discipline. When you find yourself in a low place, ask yourself these questions instead of giving up right away:

"Am I too tough on myself?" "Are adverse thoughts distorting my opinion?" "How can this setback/obstacle/failure be used to your advantage?" Why was this objective important to me? What was my goal?' "Is this purpose still important to me?" Who should I ask for help? A smart way to check in on your attitude is to ask yourself these questions. It's all too quick to get frustrated when we get caught up in negative thinking or lose sight of our intent.

Wrap Up

Learning to identify negative tendencies and take steps to correct them early with healthy habits is a vital part of improving mental toughness. It is not about removing vulnerability to improve mental toughness but learning how to cope with it and resolve it. No one is flawless, but we can grow mental toughness worthy of life's greatest challenges if we concentrate on the right stuff.

REFERENCES

Burns, C. (2015). *Instant motivation: The surprising truth behind what really drives top performance.*

Change Your Thinking, Change Your Life A Time for a Change. (2014). Archway.

Davenport, B., & Scott, S. J. (2016). *Declutter your mind: How to stop worrying, relieve anxiety, and eliminate negative thinking.* United States?: Oldtown Publishing.

Klein, G. (2004). *The power of intuition: How to use your gut feelings to make better decisions at work.* New York: Currency/Doubleday.

Landman, S. (2015). *Confidence.* New York: Brooklyn Arts Press.

Marotta, J. (2014). *50 mindful steps to self-esteem: Everyday practices for cultivating self-acceptance and self-compassion.* Oakland: New Harbinger.

Maxwell, J. C. (2016). *How successful people think: Change your thinking, change your life.* New York: Center Street.

Pigliucci, M., Cleary, S., & Kaufman, D. (2020). *How to live a good life: A guide to choosing your personal philosophy.* New York: Vintage Books/Penguin Random House LLC.

Problem solving. (2009). North Sydney, NSW: 3P Learning.

Salzgeber, N. (2017). *Stop Procrastinating: A Simple Guide to Hacking Laziness, Building Self Discipline, and Overcoming Procrastination.*

Schiraldi, G. R. (2007). *10 simple solutions for building self-esteem: How to end self-doubt, gain confidence, and create a positive self-image.* Oakland, CA: New Harbinger Publications.

Sylver, M. (1997). *Passion, profit & power: Reprogram your subconscious mind to create the relationships, wealth, and well-being that you deserve.* New York: Simon & Schuster.

www.ingramcontent.com/pod-product-compliance
Lightning Source LLC
Chambersburg PA
CBHW021437080526
44588CB00009B/566